I0118356

COMPLETE
PAIN

Forget Everything You Thought That You Knew About Pain

by
JAMES W. FORSYTHE M.D., H.M.D.

"Complete Pain ~ Forget Everything You Thought
That You Knew About Pain"

Century Wellness Publishing
521 Hammill Lane
Reno, NV 895011

Copyright © 2011, By James W. Forsythe, M.D., H.M.D.

All rights reserved, including the right of reproduction in whole
or in part in any form

Designed by Patty Atcheson-Melton, Wow Design Marketing, Inc.
&
Margie Enlow, NuDirections Graphic Design Marketing

Forsythe, M.D., H.M.D, James W.

1. Health 2. Pain 3. Oncology

NOTICE: The author of this book and of accompanying programs has used
his best efforts to prepare this publication. Please note that any person is
responsible for his or her own medical care, and no individual should ever
attempt to develop a medical diagnosis, medical prognosis and medical
treatment for himself or for herself. All patients should seek the direct
assistance of a qualified physician, medical professional or emergency
responder. The author and publisher make no representation or warranties
with respect to the accuracy, applicability, fitness, or completeness of the
contents in this book. They disclaim any warranties (express or implied), as
to the merchantability, or fitness of the text herein for any particular
purpose. The author and publisher shall in no event be held liable for any
loss or other damages, including but not limited to special, incidental, con-
sequential or other damages due to the printed contents herein.

This book/manual contains material protected under International and
Federal Copyright Laws and Treaties. Any unauthorized reprint or
use of this material is prohibited, under civil and
federal and governmental penalties.

ISBN: 978-0-9848383-1-8

DEDICATION

This "*Complete Pain*" book is dedicated to the over 50,000 patients I have treated in the past 40 years with varying degrees of pain in every anatomical site ranging from headaches to ulcerating skin cancers to pathologic fractures of bones, to deep-seated chest and intra-abdominal pelvic pains. Included in these extreme examples are the severe neuropathic pains related to neurotoxic effects of certain chemotherapy agents. From every one of these patients I have learned important lessons on the boundless courage of the human spirit.

I have seen the sincere compassion and commitment of caring family members and close friends helping to provide support and assistance in their loved-ones' extreme time of need. I have witnessed the power of prayers, love and humor to defeat the onslaught of the ravages of these often overwhelming symptoms. My heart goes out to these extraordinary families and friends who give hope, courage and selfless devotion until the end.

ACKNOWLEDGEMENT

To my good friend and literary editor and consultant Wayne Rollan Melton, a seasoned journalist and author himself who added spice and seasoning to the subject, adding a zest to this vital topic which some people would otherwise consider mundane and dreary. To Patty Melton of WOW! Design Marketing and Margie Enlow of NuDirection Design for their formatting and cover production. To my entire office staff and especially my loving wife, Earlene, for her inspiration and encouragement. To my wonderful five children and ten grandchildren who give me motivation to write.

Contents

INTRODUCTION

Life Itself is
the Essence of Pain

There would be no life at all without labor pain such as in childbirth. By some accounts, at least 255 babies are born worldwide every minute. Yet sadly, judging by statistics from the University of Queensland in Australia at least once every few minutes one new mother dies in an incidence of maternal mortality or "obstetrical death" that often results from extreme pain and the resulting complications while giving birth.

Many scientists and physicians might even go so far as to call this "natural," a calling sign of Mother Nature. After all, pain surrounds and plagues us beginning from the multi-hour period when we are born, until hitting many individuals hard again during the final moments before death. By some accounts, infants feel pain or discomfort during the birthing process. And for many senior citizens death comes as a relief, the end of pain.

Seemingly since time began poets and lyricists have expounded that "life is a bucket of tears." Indeed, the age-old adage remains only partly correct when we're told that "the only things certain in life are death and taxes." Like those outcomes, pain reigns as an inescapable and highly predictable factor throughout all of our lives as well. Just as we know with certainty that the sun will rise and set each day, physicians can reliably predict that you will suffer physical pain at every stage of life.

15

"There is no more lively sensation than that of pain," said the Marquis de Sade, a French aristocrat from the 18th and 19th Centuries credited with creating the term "sadism." "Its impressions are certain and dependable."

Both Nature and People Inflict Horrific Pain

The inescapable process that entails physical pain encompasses everything from the physical realm of our bodies to the emotional aspects of our inner psyches.

The pain that one individual suffers in the death process often ignites emotional distress in those who survive. Paradoxically, with just as much intensity some people experience extreme sensations of delight, a devilish glee upon witnessing people as they suffer excruciating pain.

Nearly 2,000 years ago at the Colosseum in Rome tens of thousands of people often cheered wildly when watching gruesome executions. Many festivities featured precise re-enactments of famous battles. The entertainment frequently involved the hunts of wild animals ranging from lions and giraffes to elephants. Today, some behavioral experts might argue that such gore extends to modern realistic-appearing video games.

Throughout history people have lusted for the blood rush of inflicting pain on others. With just as much intensity, almost all of us instinctively will go to tremendous lengths to do whatever possible to avoid pain or to eliminate such sensations after they begin. We buy tens of billions of dollars in pharmaceuticals in hopes of masking or blocking the sensation of physical pain and of emotional distress as well.

In fact, as unbelievable as this might sound, when forced to make a sudden decision many of us would choose a gruesome death rather than having to suffer intense pain. Rather than face the horrific pain of flames, at least 62 of the146 garment workers who died in the Triangle Shirtwaist Factory fire of 1909 leaped to their deaths from the eighth, ninth and tenth floors of the former Asch Building in New York City. According to at least one published account, a man and woman were seen kissing each other at a window before each jumped to their deaths to escape the flames.

"Sweet is true love that is given in vain, and sweet is death that takes away pain," said Lord Alfred Tennyson, a Poet Laureate in the United Kingdom during the 19th Century.

Society Uses Pain to Punish and to Reward

Lots of people seeking revenge insist that condemned killers should suffer as much pain as possible in the execution process. Some angry relatives of murder victims today complain that many of those condemned in the United States "have it easy" thanks to lethal injections. Some survivors tell the news media immediately after executions. "He should have suffered the way his victims did."

Whatever position each of us feels deep down in our hearts about such conflictive issues, our physical and emotional instincts tell us that pain is extremely important to the human condition. Such sensations can rule or at least play a major role in our behaviors. Yes, amid traumatic incidences, instinct tells us to take a "fight or flight" mode—either flee to avoid pain or enter battle in order to inflict suffering on others, and thereby—hopefully—escape just such a fate ourselves.

Heralded as a "doctor of death," the pathologist Jack Kevorkian claimed to have assisted at least 130 people in committing suicide in the late 20th Century. Among his primary objectives was to eliminate suffering, largely because the ravages of extreme pain experienced by these patients' due to terminal disabilities had robbed them of basic human dignity. In some cases these individuals complained of having to endure persistent and intense pain, their lives unnecessarily and even cruelly prolonged by medicines and machines well past the point of what some people consider the basic "quality of life."

Approaching the world with just as much ferocity as Kevorkian, World War II Congressional Medial of Honor recipient Audie Murphy of the U.S. Army was credited in various media accounts with killing as many as 240 German soldiers. Some sociologists might argue that Murphy took the heroic measures during several intense battles in order to "kill or be killed," an extreme measure to prevent himself and his buddies from suffering.

"There are no gains without pain," said Benjamin Franklin, a founding father of the United States, famed as a politician, statesman, scientist, diplomat and satirist.

Complicating matters, in keeping with their profession's standard and recommended protocol, many physicians must use potentially painful medications or treatments on patients in order to attempt a "cure" or at least to generate a lessening of painful symptoms. From chemotherapy for cancer to the amputation of limbs on the battle-field amid the heat of war, doctors have used what they considered the best-short term pain-reducing options.

Misconceptions About Pain Abound

Common folklore even specifies that dentists suffer from a super-high suicide rate due to the stigma of having to inflict pain upon lots of people. Many statisticians scoff at such observations, labeled as pure nonsense thrust upon a gullible public. Even so, this unfounded perception seems to persist at least in the eyes of many.

"The truth is rarely pure, and never simple," said Oscar Wilde, the widely acclaimed Irish writer and poet from the late 1800s.

Nonetheless, people from diverse cultures in many eras have looked to their individual faiths for guidance in matters involving pain. When faced with life-and-death decisions, forced to decide whether to inflect pain on others, many people choose to embrace the teachings of Jesus of Nazareth in his Sermon on the Mount. The Bible tells believers worldwide that Jesus commanded us to "turn the other cheek," and the Golden Rule of "do unto others as you would have them do unto you."

Through the millennia many of the world's most prevalent religions have given varying reasons for why humans must endure physical pain and heartache. To the Christians, as told in Genesis 3:16-17, after Adam and Eve—the world's first people—ate forbidden fruit, the Lord told them that she would suffer severe pains in childbirth forevermore, and that he would have to painfully toil for food all the days of his life.

Even from the eyes of many agnostics and to atheists, life is filled with rivers of seemingly endless pain that seems to lack any significant meaning. The 19th Century German philosopher Friedrich Nietzsche proclaimed that a "casual stroll through the lunatic asylum proves that faith does not prove anything."

For the believers and the non-believers alike, however, there are those of us who embrace statements such as those by TV and movie star Mary Tyler Moore, quoted as saying: "Pain nourishes courage. You can't be brave if you've only had wonderful things happen to you."

Herein we must come to grips with integral primordial questions that face us all, to varying degrees throughout each stage of life. What exactly is physical pain? Why must we suffer? How much should we have to endure? Why do some of us actually want to suffer physical and emotional pain, or to inflict such sensations on others?

Perhaps just as important, how much—if at all—must we watch our loved ones suffer? What reasonable and reliable measures can we take to relieve or eliminate the pain of those that we cherish? And, throughout these natural processes, how can we individually and collectively use the ravages of physical pain to our advantage?

Before grasping these integral basics, we first must seize and accept a keen understanding of the vital and essential role that pain plays in almost every aspect of our lives. Only then, enriched by this blessed knowledge, can we put our own hearts at ease while learning to control as much pain as we can—while also accepting any unmanageable hurts and aches as best as our hearts allow.

James W. Forsythe, M.D., H.M.D.

Chapter 1

Pain Can Sometimes Serve as a Blessing

No matter how much we try to think otherwise, pain can emerge as a wonderful blessing. Yes, physical pain can warn us when something has gone terribly wrong with our bodies, potentially notifying us to take necessary and decisive medical action. Emotional agony and heartache also can serve as integral signals of severe internal distress.

"Pain insists upon being attended to," said C.S. Lewis, a 20th Century novelist, literary critic, and lay theologian. "God whispers to us in our pleasures, speaks in our consciences, but shouts in our pains. It is his megaphone to rouse a deaf world."

How we respond—if at all—to the onset of physical pain invariably plays a significant role in a probable cessation of symptoms, and quite possibly a cure to an underlying problem. A timely response can make the difference between life and death, or the difference between a brief illness and a potential lifelong disability.

A wide variety of diseases and afflictions spanning from cancer to AIDS can be effectively treated, particularly when recognized and fully acknowledged in the early stages. Much of the time positive outcomes hinge on appreciating the importance of pain. For this reason, people who suffer from chronic or unexpected pain should:

- Notify: Visit a physician, medical professional or health care facility as soon as possible.

- Vigilant: Adhere to recommended or prescribed treatments without getting off track.

- Follow-Up: Schedule and keep subsequent medical appointments to track the progress of disease or injury in order to implement or modify treatments to get the best pain-relieving results.

According to many news reports, women are far more likely to get regular medical check-ups even for instances involving pain. Some medical professionals and analysts believe this occurs because men are less likely than women to want to discuss or share personal issues involving stress, emotions and depression—known potential pain triggers. The only major exception, at least by some accounts, entails matters of sexual dysfunction, instances where men often eagerly seek medical help and advice.

An age-old saying dictates that "trouble is part of your life and if you don't share it, you don't give the person who loves you a chance to love you enough." When matters of physical pain become involved, we all should love ourselves enough to seek professional help, particularly as soon as we begin suffering unexpected physical distress.

James W. Forsythe, M.D., H.M.D.

Ignoring Pain Can Result in Death

Individuals who choose to ignore pain or who flat-out refuse to seek a medical diagnosis often suffer death that might otherwise have been prevented. Many people with diseases and their relatives learn too late that those severe chest pains, jaw aches, headaches or backaches are the precursors to sudden fatalities that could have been prevented.

"Oh, don't call an ambulance," some people say in what turns out to become their final statements. "We cannot afford the bills. This must be just heartburn, or a hangover. Let's wait a little while and see if this thing passes."

Early detection, in many cases thanks to the initial onset of pain, can lead to reversal of serious medical conditions, possibly resulting in a return to good health. Statistics provided by a wide variety of health organizations indicate the definite benefits of early detection of diseases ranging from heart problems to cancer.

According to documentation provided by the American Cancer Society, "regular use of some established screening tests can prevent the development of cancer through identification and removal or treatment of pre-malignant abnormalities. Screening tests can also improve survival and decrease mortality by deleting cancer at an early stage when treatment is more effective." The society has published its annual Cancer Prevention and Early Detection Facts and Figures since 1992.

Indeed, now entering my fifth decade as a full-time oncologist, I have seen countless cases where many people failed to heed the warning signs of pain—often until after it was too late to render effective treatment. On the positive side, many patients also quickly helped put themselves on track toward a return to vibrant health by visiting my office or the

25

facilities of other medical professionals soon after initial pains began. For people suffering from chest pains or severe aches in the jaw, neck, shoulders, back or arms—particularly on the body's left side—the American Heart Association recommends getting immediate medical attention. Necessary or recommended tests during—or immediately after such episodes—include documentation of a complete medical history, a complete physical examination, an electrocardiogram and blood tests.

Besides potential heart or cancer problems, a wide range of other possible diseases that pain can signal range from the onset of arthritis, cholera, muscular ailments, malaria, the flu, lung disease, circulatory problems, Lyme disease, and many others. In many instances some of these afflictions are first noticed via the onset of pain, including numerous afflictions that can emerge as debilitating or fatal unless detected early.

Common sense dictates that all of us should heed the early warning signs of pain, rather than risk having physicians discover what we consider the worst possible outcomes. As the widely acclaimed genius Albert Einstein once proclaimed: "God does not play dice."

Even the World's Greatest Leaders Ignored Pain

Throughout history, many of the world's greatest leaders have failed to heed the notice given by the early onset of critical pain. So, if you are currently at this particular stage in your life, refrain from blaming yourself if you ignored initial pains, and now find yourself in extremely poor health as a result. Remember, we're all "only human."

Key among people who made such "mistakes" perhaps was the Father of Our Country, George Washington, the first president of the United States. During an extremely cold winter on December, 12, 1797, more than two years after his second and final term in office, Washington spent an evening on horseback amid extreme cold, freezing rain and snowfall while inspecting his farms at Mount Vernon near Alexandria, Virginia.

Immediately afterward, at age 67 Washington made the fatal mistake of ignoring the apparent pain or obvious discomfort caused by this exposure to the elements. Historians tell us that this great, brave and wise man ate dinner rather than changing out of his extremely cold and wet clothes. Washington promptly caught a severe sore throat, and the illness quickly progressed until he died two days later.

While historians might argue about the specific causes of Washington's death, at least one factor remains clear, something that we all can learn from today. Rather than merely seeking medical attention at the onset of pain, we also should take immediate action ourselves or on behalf of others in order to eliminate or lessen painful situations.

"Learn from yesterday, live for today, and hope for tomorrow," Einstein said. "The important thing is not to stop questioning."

Negative Outcomes Remain Possible

Sadly, many people who strive to take immediate and decisive action at the onset of pain also end up receiving a negative outcome or even suffering death. Sometimes the worst possible outcomes occur because physicians give improper medications for the treatment of pain. Other deaths occur when patients accidentally take lethal doses of prescribed medications.

Arguably one of the most famous of these instances involved the 1973 death in Hong Kong at age 32 of Bruce Lee, a popular movie star, martial arts instructor and philosopher. At the time many of Lee's fans considered him as perhaps the world's most highly conditioned athlete pound-for-pound. According to various news reports, Lee's bodybuilding, weight training and calisthenics placed him in a vastly superior athletic level. His speeds at performing push-ups, chin-ups and sidekicks remain legendary.

Despite Lee's superior conditioning, in May 1973 he began suffering from severe headaches and seizures. That month Lee was rushed to a Hong Kong hospital where physicians diagnosed him with cerebral edema, which occurs when excessive amounts of water accumulate within the brain. According to various reports, doctors released Lee from the hospital that month after using Mannitol, a white, crystalline organic compound to release the swelling.

News reports indicated that on July 20, 1973, Lee complained of a headache while visiting the home of a colleague, Taiwanese actress Betty Ting Pei, to discuss the production of a planned movie. Journalists reported that Pei gave Lee a standard analgesic pain reliever, Equagesic, which contained both aspirin and a muscle relaxant.

After taking this medication, Lee went to lie down for a nap but he soon failed to arrive at a restaurant for a scheduled dinner meeting with movie producer Raymond Chow. The concerned producer visited the Pei residence but was unable to awaken Lee with the assistance of a physician. Numerous reports say Lee died before they could get him to the hospital. An autopsy reported that Lee suffered from considerable brain swelling.

Twenty-seven months later Chow said in an interview that Lee had died from hypersensitivity to the muscle relaxant in Equagesic. Doctors officially listed the cause as "death by misadventure." Still another report quoted a neurosurgeon as stating that cannabis also may have played a factor.

Whatever the specific cause of Lee's death, we can and should use his tragic passing as a vital lesson. Ultimately each of us should seek treatments only from qualified physicians or medical professionals, while avoiding attempts to diagnose ourselves. And, you should never ingest a powerful medication unless a physician has prescribed that drug specifically for you. Yet, sadly, many people fail to heed such basics.

"Common sense is not so common," said Voltaire, a French writer and philosopher in the 18th Century.

Pain Motivated Celebrities to Kill Themselves

Just like countless other people have worldwide, many celebrities have chosen to commit suicide primarily in order to end physical pains that medications failed to relieve.

In 1997 at age 75, movie star Brian Keith died of a self-inflicted gunshot wound in Malibu, California, while suffering from painful emphysema and lung cancer. Chronic pain often exacerbates the perception of suffering from other personal situations. Keith's death came two months after the separate suicide of his daughter Daisy, who appeared with him in the short-lived series "Heartland" in 1989.

And according to news accounts Keith also was undergoing severe personal financial problems.

Actor Hervé Villechaize, a star of the hit ABC-TV series "Fantasy Island" from 1978 to 1984, also portrayed an evil henchman in the 1974 James Bond film, "The Man With the Golden Gun." Villechaize died at age 50 in 1993 of a self-inflicted gunshot wound, leaving a note describing his despondency that resulted from longtime health problems. Villechaize's dwarfism apparently caused extremely severe physical pain, a common symptom suffered by many middle-aged people with this condition. Such symptoms sometimes lead to chronic depression like those that he reportedly suffered.

In 1999, actor Richard Farnsworth finished filming his starring role in the critically acclaimed film "The Straight Story," for which he received an Oscar® nomination for best actor. During production, Farnsworth suffered from extremely severe pain caused by bone cancer, which may have been the result of prostate cancer that he began suffering in the early 1990s. Rather than live the remainder of his life in severe physical pain, Farnsworth fatally shot himself at his Lincoln, New Mexico, ranch on Oct. 6, 2000.

The deaths of Keith, Villechaize and Farnsworth mark just a handful of the seemingly countless suicides by celebrities and common everyday people worldwide, often carried out with the primary intent of relief from physical pain. Seemingly every day it seems that people choose this ultimate decision to end their own lives for this very reason.

"To run away from trouble is a form of cowardice," said Aristotle, the famed Greek philosopher from the fourth century before Christ. "And, while it is true that the suicide braves death, he does it not for some noble object but to escape some ill."

James W. Forsythe, M.D., H.M.D.

Pain Leads to Other Severe Conditions

Besides suicide, chronic and debilitating physical pain often leads to a wide variety of extremely severe mental and physical conditions. Key among these is chronic depression, a mental disorder called by a wide variety of names. People suffering from severe physical pain sometimes experience some of the worst symptoms or attributes of chronic depression.

Often suffering so much physical pain that they become disabled, those experiencing chronic depression sometimes lose their sense of self worth. A common complaint involves an inability to seek or experience pleasure.

When this occurs, virtually everything in a person's lifestyle is impacted. Chronic depression adversely impacts family life, the ability to effectively interact with other individuals, and the ability to perform or achieve basic goals at school or at work.

"The term clinical depression finds its way into too many conversations these days," said Leonard Cohen, a Canadian novelist, poet and musician. "One has a sense that a catastrophe has occurred in the psychic landscape."

Despite such observations, there is no denying that chronic depression is an extremely serious condition that can lead to a variety of negative physical conditions. Such situations often adversely impact all vital aspects of generally good health, ranging from sleeping and eating habits to the lack of a healthy sex life.

Exacerbating matters, certain pharmaceuticals that are administered in hopes of alleviating or masking the effects of physical pain

31

sometimes lead to mood disorders. Also compounding the problem, these difficulties can potentially worsen to the point that the immune system weakens, leading to or increasing the probability of severe infections.

Faced with such extreme potential outcomes, patients and physicians find themselves challenged by the need to face physical pain and its causes head-on. Only through such direct efforts can effective results occur. The ultimate goal always remains the total elimination or the masking of physical pain, thereby opening up a pathway toward potential happiness or at least the resumption of average, common lifestyles.

"To enjoy good health, to bring true happiness to one's family, to bring peace to all, one must first discipline and control one's own mind," said the Buddha, a spiritual teacher and the founder of Buddhism in about the fifth century before Christ. "If a man can control his mind, he can find the way to enlightenment, and all wisdom and virtue will naturally come to him."

Chapter 2

Good News ~ Find Hope to Relieve Pain

W hile all these essential statistics might seem depressing from the start, good news awaits people who remain determined to escape the ravages of pain. A time-tested variety of behavior strategies, pharmaceutical regimens, and natural homeopathic herbs benefit individuals willing to learn and implement these various methods.

Herein you will discover the essential techniques, many little-known and rarely mentioned in the mainstream media in any helpful in-depth manner. Adding luster to these lessons, many of the best pain-relieving tools or lifestyles cost little or nothing to put into action. The key to success often hinges on first learning the basics.

Those who stand to benefit range from people severely debilitated by crippling arthritis to individuals suffering severe pains ranging from cancer, chemotherapy, kidney stones, childbirth labor, toothaches and many other ailments. Throughout this process, you'll also learn time-tested strategies for avoiding the potential danger of becoming addicted to extreme, life-altering addictions to painkillers.

"Hope is important because it can make the present moment less difficult to bear," said Nhat Hanh, a poet, Buddhist monk, teacher and author. "If we believe that tomorrow will be better, we can bear a hardship today."

Among the many systems that you will soon learn in order to sharply increase the probability of putting your life back into a manageable mode:

- The Ladder of Pain Control: The best, time-tested system of increasing or decreasing the intensity of pain-blocking pharmaceuticals and natural remedies.

- Mind control: Techniques recommended for several millenniums by master physicians, relaxing the mind and body to lessen the impact of pain.

- Natural substances: Numerous natural substances rarely mentioned in the mainstream media, but proven as highly effective in eliminating severe aches.

- Peace of mind: A mixture in varying degrees of one or more of these techniques, partly in order to prevent the possibility of extreme mental depression.

- Symptom prevention: Unique, creative and little-known strategies for stopping potential pain dead in its tracks before such hassles even have a chance to begin.

Long before the advent of today's standard allopathic medicines, people from various cultures used effective pain-killing methods rarely employed in today's western world. For many of us, the key to avoiding unnecessary standard drugs is to first employ one or more of several relatively safe, non-invasive methods for eliminating or preventing physical pain. In fact, in many cases the greatest successes emerge for individuals who consider this process an all-out, intense war against such physical conditions.

Make no little plans—they have no magic to stir men's blood and probably will not themselves be realized," said Daniel H. Burnham, an architect and urban planner in the late 19th Century and early 20th Century. "Make big plans; aim high in hope and work, remembering that a noble, logical diagram once recorded will not die."

This especially holds true for anyone, even you, who happens to now suffer from debilitating, life-wrecking pain. So, from the start each of us first needs to know the essential basics of pain, exactly how and why this sensation occurs within the body.

The Good, the Bad and the Ugly Details of Pain

"Pain is good because it's bad," Dr. Anne Louise Oaklander, a pain specialist once told NBC News. "And it's the badness, the unpleasantness; the horrible emotions that are evoked when we feel pain that make it work so well."

Some patients who suffer from severe limb injuries from car accidents tell physicians that the pain feels as if they're being stabbed with knives and needles. People who have been shot often describe the sensation that seemed as if getting stabbed by thunderbolts.

These sensations become possible only because physical receptors connected to nerves throughout the body communicate the information to the spinal cord. From there, the information shoots up into the brain, the organ that actually gives us the sensation of "feeling pain."

In a sense, for instance, when you stub your toe on furniture in a dark room during the middle of the night, the actual sensation of pain is not in your foot but inside your brain.

This remains a critical and essential point to remember, especially for anyone interested in immediately counteracting or eliminating the uncomfortable sensations of pain.

A key to the process of your body expressing the sensation of pain are peripheral nerves leading through the spinal cord. Peripheral nerves detect problems in essential areas of the body, including the skin, internal organs, muscles, joints and bones. The endings of peripheral nerves are extremely sensitive, capable of discerning between the subtle differences of touch, temperature variations, vibrations, pressures and severe injury.

Among the peripheral nerves are nociceptors that serve as the body's essential and vital sensory receptors that detect potentially severe internal damage or injuries. Physicians call this process "nociception," the integral and important trigger of perceiving pain.

We Would Die Without Suffering Pain

Like all mammals, humans would literally die unless they "possessed the ability to suffer" from physical pain, especially because that sensation commands that we take action to address the problem.

Imagine suffering from a severed hand in a car accident. Any such person who is otherwise healthy, and retains or regains consciousness obviously experiences excruciating pain. Those capable of tending to their own wound likely would do so or attempt to seek the help of others as soon as possible. To ignore such a wound could very likely result in gangrene, hemorrhage or even death.

All areas of the body except the face contain essential dorsal root ganglions, interconnected to the spinal nerve system and relaying sensory information to the brain. The information transmission process from the site of an injury or disease to the head amazes even experienced medical professionals.

The nerve ending within the face that detect pain is the trigeminal ganglion, part of the fifth cranial nervous system. These nerves are essential in the eating, speaking, eye movement, and smelling processes. Anyone who has ever accidentally bitten his tongue while eating or been hit in the face has learned first-hand the super-sensitivity of this nervous system.

Boxing athlete Randall "Tex" Cobb has been quoted as saying that "if you screw things up in tennis, it's 15-love. If you screw things up in boxing, it's your ass."

Your Brain Welcomes Sensations of Pain

After initial transmission from nociceptors, the nerve fibers within the spinal cord send the information about pain upward toward the brain. The dorsal horn serves as the location where peripheral nerves enter the spinal cord. In order to transmit their signals, the nerve fibers release neurotransmitters. These electrical signals strive to activate various nerve cells, which work to convey the information to the thalamus within the brain's midportion.

Located between the midbrain and the cerebral cortex, the thalamus works to regulate a variety of functions including sleep, consciousness and alertness. The thalamus also regulates or detects a sense of space, and various physical sensations including pain.

As soon as the thalamus receives communication about pain, it forwards this information to three separate areas of the brain. They are:

- The Somatosensory cortex: Located in the upper center of the brain called the parietal lobe, this identifies and detects the degree and location of pain within the body.

- Limbic system: This consists of a set of various structures within the brain above the brain stem, which work together to elicit emotion regarding the pain signals.

- The frontal lobe: Sometimes referred to as the frontal cortex, this area is often referred to as the "thinking" part of the brain. It can assign "meaning" to signals of pain, while pondering— and eventually deciding—what actions to take.

Whenever possible, the brain also orders the body to begin producing natural pain killers called endorphins and enkephalins. Endorphins often generate pleasant natural sensations, generated by the body when a person exercises, experiences love, enjoys orgasms, feels excitement, tastes spicy foods, or experiences physical pain.

In essence, when you suffer from a serious injury or disease, Mother Nature strives to make you feel the physical pain and to experience emotion that serves as a call to action—while also striving to make you ponder possible solutions.

"If the mortality rate seems high we must realize that nature is a ruthless teacher," said William S. Burroughs, a 20th Century American novelist, poet and essayist. "There are no second chances in Mother Nature's survival course."

Consider the Three Primary Pain Remedies

A combination of modern technology, nature and age-old remedies give us three primary strategies or short-term fixes for addressing physical pain. They are:

- Message blocking: Various pharmaceuticals and natural products that work to block the nerve system's messaging system, preventing the brain from recognizing pain.

- Health renewal: Curing or fixing the body's area that has been wounded in accidents or attacks, or specific organs afflicted by disease, or the primary illness.

- Mind control and prevention: Training the mind to block perceptions of pain, or adopting lifestyles or physical devices that are likely to prevent or lessen the likelihood of painful conditions.

Huge portions of the entire medical profession are designed to bring out the best possible results in each of these strategies. Since pain or the lack of it plays an integral role in our health, significant emphasis is placed on these methods. By some estimates many hundreds of billions or perhaps trillions of dollars are spent yearly on pain-relief.

And yet amazingly, despite significant advances in the practice of medicine, physicians still lack a single cure-all method of preventing or eliminating physical pain. Even since early childhood, many of us began hearing that common phrase, "there is no cure for the common cold." But few people pay attention to the fact medicine also lacks a single, reliable and predictably effective, non-addictive cure for excruciating physical pain.

Complete Pain

In matters involving pain some people embrace and adhere to the longstanding lifestyle theme that "ignorance is bliss," since the mere thought of suffering with—and the seeking remedies for—severe pain seems extremely difficult or even insurmountable.

Others facing pain embrace action-oriented strategies such as those stressed by the late 20th Century civil rights activist the Rev. Dr. Martin Luther King Jr., who said, "Nothing in this world is more dangerous than a sincere ignorance and conscientious stupidity."

Chapter 3

More Good News ~ Most Physical Pain is Manageable

 For those learning the basic intricacies that involve physical pain, good news emerges when they discover that most cases by far are short-term and easily medicated.

On a regular or seemingly consistent basis almost everyone has suffered from common everyday cuts, bruises, sprains, blisters, headaches and joint aches. Remember that pain hails as a basic fact of life, and to satisfy the public's need to address minor afflictions, pharmaceutical and medical supply companies have developed a plethora of materials and over-the-counter drugs.

According to some estimates, the average American family spends about $185 yearly on non-prescription remedies. This brings the nationwide total for such purchases to many tens of billions of dollars.

The overall dollar totals catapult to far greater levels when accounting for prescription medications that only licensed doctors can legally administer, at least when distribution is handled on a domestic basis. Estimates vary widely, partly because significant numbers of Americans strive to buy pharmaceuticals cheaply online from international suppliers, rather than pay exorbitant U.S. prices.

The failure of the medical industry to develop a single affordable, reliable and predictable method of eliminating severe pain has played a primary role in driving up prices for essential prescription-based painkillers and other essential pharmaceuticals. In fact, the AARP, commonly known as the American Association of Retired Persons, has concluded that prescription drug prices have shot up far higher than the inflation rate.

Frustrated, angered and even left feeling hopeless due to this critical distribution system, many people repeat this commonly used observation—"Only in America do drugstores make the sick walk all the way to the back of the store to get their prescriptions, while healthy people can buy cigarettes at the front of the store."

Chronic Pain Emerges
Amid the Confusion

Amid the confusion and complexities of obtaining reliable and affordable medications for common, easily cured medical problems, some patients experience chronic pain.

Unlike regular everyday common pains that are often short-term and easily treatable, chronic pain emerges as persistent, almost never-ending and in some cases even life-threatening in nature. Compounding these problems, as an overall profession physicians lack a single, precise and universal definition of what comprises "chronic pain."

For the most part, many medical professionals seem to agree that diagnosing chronic pain becomes necessary when such symptoms persist at least three months or perhaps even six months without letup.

However, adding to the confusion among medical professionals, some physicians insist the condition of chronic pain can occur in durations of less than 30 days.

Adding to the frustration for patients, some doctors even consider chronic pain as any condition where suffering persists without letup past the expected recovery period.

Such varying and diverse—sometimes conflicting—definitions can emerge as important, largely because physicians need to adjust prescription medications and overall treatment methods, largely depending on the projected duration of a specific medical condition.

This factor emerges as critical, since insufficient levels of medications could fail to lessen or eliminate unnecessary suffering, perhaps even the weakening of a patient's immune system, thereby worsening his or her overall condition. Conversely, giving too much pain-relief medication might result in various adverse conditions, such as preventing the body's ability to naturally heal or even increasing the probability of an addiction to painkillers.

Complications such as these tend to "wear down" some patients, thereby forcing them to lose hope for a full recovery, or providing the person with a potential pathway to gradually begin to make negative lifestyle decisions regarding everyday care.

"Our fatigue is often caused not by work, but by worry, frustration and resentment," said Dale Carnegie, a 20th Century American author and lecturer who developed a widely acclaimed system for self-improvement.

For some patients, especially those suffering from chronic pain, feelings of frustration and resentment grow after various long-term treatments all fail to give relief from pain. Ultimately, largely because they lack essential and integral knowledge on the topic, many patients find themselves relying on the advice and prescriptions given by their personal physicians or medical professionals. Yet some doctors give vastly different treatments, generating situations where achieving positive results emerges as a "hit or miss" proposition.

Another Form of Pain Complicates Matters

Besides standard, typical or even severe pains that are recognized and transmitted to the brain by the body's nociceptive nerves, another unique form of pain sometimes occurs.

Neuropathic pain erupts when the nervous system suffers damage or malfunctions. This condition sometimes occurs as a result of physical injuries, or perhaps even from the ravages of disease such as cancer.

In many cases of neuropathic pain, the patient describes feeling hurt in an area of the body other than where the wound or disease occurred. This sometimes happens because specific or widespread sections of the overall nervous system have been severely damaged. Generally, physicians list neuropathic pain into two categories. They are:

- Superficial Somatic: Sometimes described as "deep pain" or deep somatic pain, these occur when nociceptors transmit sensations of poorly localized, dull or aching pains from muscles, ligaments, bones, tendons, blood vessels and other areas.

- Visceral Pain: These unwelcome sensations emanate from the organs, but physicians often have difficulty locating a specific site. Patients sometimes describe these sensations as "pins and needles," or stabbing, burning, electrical or tingling.

Meantime, neuropathic pain is transmitted to the brain via either of two sections of the nervous system. One involves the central nervous system originating from the spinal cord and brain. And the other encompasses the peripheral nervous system, emanating from areas of the body unprotected by the blood-brain barrier, skull, or spine. The blood-brain barrier is an area separate from the central nervous system.

For lay people matters involving neuropathic pain might seem complex and difficult to understand, these specific variations can emerge as important to physicians and particularly to patients seeking the most effective treatments.

Consider Pain as a Symptom Rather Than a Condition

For the most part, pain emerges only as a symptom of one or more medical conditions. In summary, as unbelievable as this might sound, pain is not the underlying problem or root cause of an original debilitating medical condition. Instead, this sensation occurs as a result of a specific biological problem such as a disease, heart attack a wound, or a physical or chemical injury.

Except for instances where the nervous system or areas of the brain are damaged, the instances where a person naturally fails to feel pain include:

- Unconsciousness: A patient is rendered unconscious, to the point where he or she fails to realize that pain is occurring. Sometimes comas occur naturally as the body's way of blocking pain, so that the organs can heal. For this reason, especially for certain cases involving severe injury, physicians sometimes intentionally induce comas in order to provide for a pain-free period for the body's natural restoration and healing processes to work.

- Death: Some or all of a particular appendage, limb or organ dies along with any sections of the nervous system within that area. Heart attacks usually result in the death of certain sections of that organ, and gangrene can kill large or small areas of the body. Frostbite also can kill peripheral areas of the body, while leaving other areas relatively healthy or intact.

With all these considerations in mind, after initially taking short-term measures to relieve pain upon seeing a new patient for the first time, many physicians immediately seek to locate and cure the underlying or primary condition that causes the discomfort.

"This is only going to hurt a little," some medical professionals such as dental assistants tell patients, immediately before rendering shots containing pain-blocking substances. Sometimes, such statements are a "lie," because these injections may create extreme discomfort that soon dissipates when the local anesthetic takes effect.

James W. Forsythe, M.D., H.M.D.

Severe Pain Can Contribute to Shock
That Results in Death

Although pain is a symptom rather than an underlying medical condition, the sensation can play a potential role in severe circulatory failure—potentially resulting in imminent or sudden death.

Along with the potentially fatal loss of blood or the loss of vital organs, people who suffer from traumatic injuries such as car wrecks or battle wounds face the possibility of circulatory shock—commonly known as "shock"—a life threatening condition that refers to a blood pressure less than 80.

In some of these critical medical events, extreme pain ravages individuals who remain partially or fully conscious. Amid or shortly following such events, the sudden elimination of pain via the use of narcotics such as morphine can help play a significant role in enabling medical professionals or battlefield medics to stabilize a patient's overall medical condition. This sometimes opens a pathway for additional treatments and, hopefully, eventual recovery.

Physicians have chronicled many types of circulatory shock, almost all of them potentially fatal. These range from septic shock that involves the loss of blood circulation from bacterial infection to vital organs and to hypovolaemic shock that occurs due to extreme blood loss and falling blood pressure.

Circulatory shock can lead to various life-ending events or conditions, such as cardiac arrest where the heart stops and hypoxemia where arterial blood fails to receive a necessary and essential supply of oxygen.

"Well, the tragedy is over," said Albert Camus, a 20th Century French Algerian journalist, philosopher and author. "The failure is complete. I turn my head and go away. I took my share of this fight for the impossible."

Chapter 4

Discover the Mysteries of Phantom Pain

Since at least the 1500s, physicians have heard patients complain of perceived pain in areas where limbs have been severed or extremeties removed. The lay public often refers to such instances as "phantom limb pain."

Besides phantom limb sensations, medical professionals from many cultures have documented cases where patients also describe "phantom limb sensations." These people get sensations that all or portions of their missing limbs remain attached to their bodies.

According to some accounts, American neurologist Silas Weir Mitchell chronicled the existence of phantom limbs in 1871, writing that "thousands of spirit limbs were haunting as many good soldiers, (and) every now and then tormenting them."

Some startled or mystified patients insisted that the existence of their missing but still-felt limbs seemed real to them, feeling as if having the same mass and weight as any remaining appendages.

"I do believe in ghosts," said Devon Joseph Werkheiser, an American actor and writer. "Freaky things will happen, and I'm like, 'The wind didn't do that. Some spirit did.'"

Although the phenomenon of phantom pain and phantom limbs might seem otherworldly, medical professionals insist they have developed logical and conclusive findings that show these attributes exist—at least in the minds of certain patients.

Nonetheless, judging by some accounts, physicians have yet to develop a universally accepted theory on how and why these sensations occur. In any case, the prevalence of and similarities among such cases persist. The phenomena also sometimes involve people who have only portions of certain limbs due to birth defects.

Some physicians believe these varying sensations develop within the peripheral, spinal or central nervous system areas. Adding to the mystery, researchers also have insisted that the thalamus, the cortex and the body's limbic system of various structures and processes within the brain can essentially make the patient believe that a missing limb still exists.

Ultimately, in many of these cases physicians sometimes find themselves faced with the need to eliminate their patients' sensations of pain in limbs that no longer exist. Some doctors have gone so far as to prescribe pain-reducing medications, or even antidepressants or drugs used to control epileptic seizures. These efforts occasionally have generated some success.

Some Sufferers of Phantom Limbs Employ a Unique Treatment

Desperate for effective relief, some patients suffering from persistent phantom limb pain have undergone what physicians call specialized "mirror box" treatments.

From the view of many researchers, a percentage of these patients perceive pain in phantom limbs that remain clinched, at least from the perceptions of their own minds. But since the limbs do not exist, the patients are unable to naturally unclench muscles of the missing limbs—a process that people with all their appendages often use to eliminate cramps or muscular discomfort.

Some researchers think that the brain gradually starts believing that the missing limb remains intact. All along, however, the brain also incorrectly senses on occasion that the phantom appendage fails to send messages due to apparent paralysis. To correct this problem, some medical professionals strive to give the brain visual feedback via the "mirror box" process, thereby creating an impression that the limb has moved.

Medical professionals occasionally use mirrors in order to develop this desired visual impression, thereby creating an image that the missing limb still exists. Upon seeing this image live in a mirror, the patient is instructed to send motor or mental orders to the missing limb and to the remaining opposite limb to make symmetric or similar movements. The objective is to make the brain believe that the missing limb has actually moved, while no longer paralyzed.

In a sense, at least to casual observers, it would seem that medical professionals need to emulate the role of magicians, to switch the brain into a recovery mode via the use of visual trickery or at least creating false illusions.

"In the many years that I have been before the public, my secret methods have been steadily shielded," said Harry Houdini, an American magician and stunt performer whose popularity crested in the early 20th Century. The magic secrets "have been shielded by the strict integrity of my assistants, most of whom have been with me for years."

Unlike such entertainers, medical professionals can and should continue to share their various successes in order to develop the most effective treatment methods.

Use the Mind as a Powerful Weapon Against Pain

When treating pain, we should remain cognizant that the great power of our minds, and of our individual personal belief systems are formidable. Many important or famous events throughout history tell us that some people have used the strength of their minds to literally ignore or persevere despite potentially excruciating or debilitating physical pain.

One of the most famous of these incidents involved Rasputin, a Russian mystic in the early 20th Century. Widely acclaimed for his formidable willpower, and his vastly superior abilities as a healer and prophet, Rasputin survived a 1914 assassination attempt where a woman stabbed him in the abdomen. This wound temporarily left his entrails protruding from his body, until surgeons repaired the injury.

Thereafter, at least according to Rasputin's daughter, he regularly took opium to relieve his pain. Yet that substance never played a role in his eventual and still legendary 1916 murder. According to at least one account, within the confines of a cellar a team of assassins tricked this mystic into eating several cyanide-laced cakes that failed to cause him any significant harm or pain.

Worried that the poisons seemed to fail, one of the assassins ran upstairs, retrieved a revolver and fired a shot through Rasputin's back. After the mystic fell, the assassins left, but according to various accounts one of them returned to the cellar to get his coat. But the famed Rasputin, sometimes known as "the mad monk," suddenly opened his eyes and lunged at the man.

According to some published reports, despite having eaten several poison-laced cakes and being shot in the back, Rasputin was able to start strangling the man—whispering into his ear, "you bad boy." Just then the assassins returned, shortly before firing three more shots into the mystic's back.

Some accounts insist that Rasputin fell once again but remained alive, even as the assailants clubbed the mystic and sexually mutilated him. Determined to finish their job, the assassins then wrapped Rasputin's body in a carpet and threw him into the Neva River where he broke free from the bindings but drowned.

The tale of Rasputin's death is but one of the countless instances where people have used their own positive thinking and the force of their own will to survive much longer than expected and to ultimately endure despite excruciating pain. These many remarkable instances can serve as a reminder to seriously ill people that largely through willpower they can endure.

"God has seen your tears and heard your prayers," Rasputin once said, while treating Russian Tsar's Nicholas II's son, Alexei, as the child recovered from an extremely serious episode of hemophilia. "Fear not, the child will not die."

Many People Have Survived Excruciating Pain

Anyone suffering from extreme pain today can take at least some comfort in knowing that many people have survived severe discomforts before returning to good health.

On Dec. 7, 2007, a 37-year-old window washer plummeted 47 stories on a scaffolding that became disengaged from a Manhattan skyscraper. According to news accounts, Alcides Moreno suffered from many broken bones throughout his entire body. Thanks to modern medical techniques physicians strived to control Moreno's pain, while successfully performing multiple surgeries.

Moreno's brother Edgar had died in the same accident. Thanks largely to his own determination coupled with the moral and professional support of his surviving family members and physicians, Alcides Moreno was soon on track for a full recovery. In January 2008, doctors announced that Moreno would regain his ability to walk.

While many people worldwide considered Moreno's recovery as miraculous, his case also serves as a prime example of how patients and physicians can successfully work together to overcome the ravages of extreme pain, injuries or disease.

In fact, any time a physician tells you to "get your affairs in order" because there is no hope of eliminating your physical pain and that same medical professional also tells you that there is "no hope of survival," you should immediately find a new doctor.

"He is the best physician who is the most ingenious inspirer of hope," said Samuel Taylor Coleridge, a 19th Century English philosopher, poet and literary critic.

Find Inspiration from Those Who Persevered

Wrapped in heavy fog on July 28, 1945, a B-25 Mitchell Bomber aircraft smashed into the 79th and 80th floors of the Empire State Building in New York City. The pilot, Lt. Col. William Franklin Smith Jr., was killed instantly, and 13 other people also perished.

The impact caused an elevator to plummet 75 floors. But miraculously the elevator operator, Betty Lou Oliver, survived despite extreme injuries that obviously caused her excruciating pain.

The accident still holds the Guinness World Record as the longest fall of an elevator that anyone has survived. The elevator cables had snapped during the rescue process, causing the device to fall into the building's basement. According to various news accounts and historic reports, Oliver returned to her job five months after the accident, winning praise from many people for her "guts" and her indomitable will to survive.

Indeed, even in the face of severe pain and extreme physical hardship, human beings possess the capability of persevering in extremely harsh conditions.

Now entering my fifth decade as a practicing oncologist, through the years I have seen numerous incidences where patients were enduring the most advanced levels of cancer pain when they were first seen.

In a number of those cases despite extreme and intense non-stop pain, some of these patients remained increasingly hopeful before eventually enjoying full and complete remission from the disease. As the disease disappears the accompanying pain also goes away.

The human spirit, the gumption to tell ourselves "never give up," can play an integral role in helping to push the body past the point of pain into the realm of full recovery.

"Victory at all cost," said Winston Churchill, prime minister of Great Britain on two separate occasions in the 20th Century—most famously during World War II. "Victory in spite of all terror, victory however long and hard the road may be, for without victory there is no survival."

Chapter 5
Fill Yourself with the Will to Survive

The will to survive, to achieve and to prosper in good health reigns as powerful and as persistent as the basic necessity of experiencing physical pain.

During the 20th Century the world-famous American daredevil Evel Knievel suffered at least 37 broken bones in various accidents. According to the Guinness Book of World Records, Knievel held the world record for the most broken bones suffered in a lifetime.

Despite horrible pain from a continuous succession of motorcycle stunt accidents, Knievel always strived to go faster and farther in his spectacular jumps. Often risking extreme pain and even death, he wanted to excel at entertaining his many fans.

Only highly trained athletic professionals should even consider attempting such fetes. All along, those of us now suffering from severe pain can embrace Knievel's strategy of striving to put such worries out of our minds.

"I forget all the things that I have broke," said Knievel, who died at age 69 of a pulmonary condition in 2007 in Clearwater, Florida. To many people Knievel's courage and winning attitude were almost heavenly in nature, perhaps the same type of spiritual, can-do attitude that patients should adopt today when striving to endure severe pain.

"Every time they wanted me to jump further, and further, and further," Knievel said. "Hell, they thought my bike had wings."

Have Faith That You Can Beat Pain

For countless generations people from many cultures have embraced that age-old adage proclaiming that "faith can move mountains."

As a practicing oncologist, homeopath and a Christian, I have personally witnessed many instances where people have used their personal, spiritual and religious faith in beating the so-called odds. At least to some degree what the masters say essentially holds true, that each of us ultimately becomes what we think we are.

If you consider yourself as whipped, a loser and beaten down forever by pain, you likely will evolve into just such a person. Conversely, those of us who strive to put ourselves in a positive, peaceful and pain-free light often find ourselves in just such a position.

As the writer Patrick Overton once proclaimed, "When you have come to the edge of all light that you know and are about to drop off into the darkness of the unknown, faith is knowing one of two things will happen—there will be something solid to stand on, or you will be taught to fly."

Certainly faith remains an essential medicine for patients suffering from pain, perhaps just as important in many cases as the various pharmaceuticals and treatments that a physician might prescribe. To ignore any possibility of embracing faith is essentially the equivalent of slapping the possibility of potential recovery clean across the face.

"You block your dream when you allow your fear to grow bigger than your faith," said Mary Manin Morrissey, a minister in Oregon.

Faithful People Truly Believe in Victory over Pain

Filled with faith that they can whip the ravages of pain and illness, every year more than 5 million people hailed as pilgrims visit the small town of Lourdes, France—which has a population of only 15,000. There, the faithful visit the Sanctuary of Our Lady of Lourdes, where believers say that Mary the Mother of Jesus made numerous visits in 1858 to Saint Marie Bernarde-Soubirous when she was only 14 years old.

At least 67 miraculous healings generated by the water at the sanctuary have been officially recorded by the Roman Catholic Church. Officials who reviewed these cases insisted that they were unable to find any psychological or physical reason for why these cures occurred, other than to conclude that "miracles" had happened.

For believers and perhaps some non-believers alike, this shrine has generated much curiosity and thereby has inspired significant hope. From my personal view, the vast majority of human beings desperately want to believe in something significant. People yearn to know and to realize within their hearts and deep inside their souls that their physical and emotional pains can and will be permanently eradicated.

Some scientists insist the water of Lourdes lacks any medicinal qualities whatsoever. And, at least judging by some widespread published accounts, the water also lacks any provable curing powers. Even so, those who believe in the miracles that occurred at the sanctuary still consider the water as an enduring symbol of faith and hope.

Certainly, any attempt to rob people of their faith in cures and that pain can be eliminated would be worse—at least in a sense—than trying to steal millions of dollars in gold from them. To the interminable human spirit, hope and faith are more precious than all the riches that our physical world could possibly provide.

"Be not afraid of life," said James Truslow Adams, a 20th Century American writer and historian. "Believe that life is worth living, and your belief will help create the fact."

Faith Fights Pain in Many Cultures

Yearning to fight pain, cure illness and to remain filled with inspirational hope, people from many cultures throughout history have flocked to those who gave them reason for faith.

In recent years various TV shows including "Oprah" and "60 Minutes" have chronicled treks by people worldwide to see a healer in Brazil. Commonly known as "John of God," João Teixeira de

Faria works as a medium and self-described "psychic surgeon" based in the state of Goiás' small town of Abadiânia.

According to published reports, João and his 30 spirit doctors claim to cure a wide variety of ailments including AIDS, tumors, asthma, cancer, blindness and the physical pains associated with these various maladies. Reported treatments range from prescription pills to surgery and medication. Some journalists report that João sometimes enters rooms filled with patients before declaring to them all that "you are cured."

Numerous patients have insisted that João cured them of a variety of ailments ranging from Lou Gehrig 's disease to brain tumors. Yet skeptics abound, many of them claiming that the supposed cures were merely a result of placebo effect, wishful thinking, conventional medicine obtained elsewhere, or "spontaneous remission"—a lay term for any unexpected and unexplainable reversal of disease and its associated pain.

Meantime, illusionists and people who investigate con artists insist that they are able to identify and expose so-called psychic surgeries performed at João's healing center, Casa de Dom Inácio de Loyola.

Whether the positive results are actual or merely perceived, there is little denying that once people get sparked by faith and hope that reliable cures exist for pain and ailments, they will do almost anything possible to obtain such treatments.

Chapter 6

My Medical Clinic Attracts Streams of People from Around the World

Many of them blessed with faith and filled with hope, each week people from around the world travel to my West Coast medical clinic. Members of my professional medical staff and my front-line employees tell me they're amazed by the continually growing number of patients. Many of these visitors first heard of me via word-of-mouth or various news media reports.

Others initially learned of my work to fight pain and disease through my various books, including one of my popular publications co-authored by media personality, actress and author Suzanne Somers. Needless to say, I feel humbled and honored every time various celebrities and many people worldwide eagerly endorse my clinics and various books.

From my view, the increasing popularity of my medical efforts stems from the methods I use to help fight pain plus the underlying ailments that ignite such symptoms. Besides the elimination of pain, patients visiting my clinic seek treatment for a wide variety of medical conditions ranging from cancer to immune disorders and general health issues.

Following 40 years in medical practice, I finally decided to generate this publication about physical pain at the urging of my many patients. Lots of these people can be seen in videos on my Website—DrForsythe.com—giving unsolicited personal heart-felt testimonials. The successful elimination of pain often hails as a primary topic.

I never seek fame or to win popularity contests. Instead, my focus remains on establishing good health and well being for my many patients, largely in hopes of relieving them of persistent pain and suffering.

Behind the scenes and with no publicity whatsoever, my office staff often gets contacted by various celebrities seeking treatment for themselves, their relatives or friends. Without exaggeration, my clinic's phones literally have been ringing almost non-stop in recent years.

"But why?" You might ask. "What makes you so special, Doctor Forsythe, that so many countless people from around the world would look to you for answers and for treatment? How are you so unique, when compared to other physicians?"

I Get Pleasure from Helping Patients

At present, I'm one of only a handful of integrative medical oncologists in the United States and from throughout the world as well. An integrative medical oncologist is a fully licensed and certified medical professional who specializes in using standard allopathic medicines to treat cancer—plus non-traditional "natural" medicines such as herbs and vitamin treatments as well.

Like almost every other typical citizen, I become disturbed and highly concerned upon seeing other human beings suffer the ravages of crippling pain. During my first several decades in practice, I primarily used standard methods accepted by allopathic physicians when implementing cancer treatments. This typically meant the use of standard chemotherapy techniques, which invariably caused my patients to suffer extensive pain.

Besides the extensive decreases in body weight and the loss of hair, many cancer patients during the early part of my career died after courageously undergoing these horrific chemotherapy treatment regimens. Mirroring nationwide statistics at the time, only an extremely small percentage—slightly more than 2 percent—of my most advanced cancer patients survived for five years early in my career.

Determined to reverse these outcomes, during the mid- and late 1990s, I also became a certified and licensed homeopath. Such medical professionals specialize in natural treatments such as herbs, rather than standard drugs that often cause or fail to alleviate what I personally consider unnecessary and excessive pain—at least in some cases.

When integrating standard-practice medicines with natural holistic or homeopathic treatments, I found that the overall survival rates of my cancer patients dramatically increased. As the years progressed, I developed specific and specialized treatments to address pain, while also fine-tuning various regimens designed to target specific types of cancers and various other diseases. My program has been called the "Forsythe Immune Therapy" or "FIT," and encompasses all the modalities that I use.

Now entering my early70s, I'm more energized and enthusiastic than ever about my medical practice, particularly the elimination of pain and the treatment of various diseases. At this stage in life, some people might think that I would want to retire in comfort, passing the proverbial baton to the next generation of physicians.

But my professional spirit and heart remain as fully energized and as enthusiastic as when I first entered the profession as an intern in the mid-1960s. The unique and continually updated methods that we're developing today are working wonders, from the view of many patients—lots of them appreciative that their pain has been lessened or eliminated much faster and with greater effectiveness than they had expected.

Some Standard Physicians Disapprove of My Efforts

Amazingly, some standard allopathic physicians and neurologists disapprove of my professional efforts. Perhaps some of their displeasure stems from simple jealousy. For the most part, though, these doctors dislike the fact that I have been widely hailed as a maverick of sorts—someone willing to "rock the boat" for the betterment of patients.

All along, a key objective in my efforts has been the effective treatment of pain. Although many people describe my practice as highly successful in this regard, lots of standard-practice doctors have worked behind the scenes in hopes of discrediting my good name.

For the most part, these medical professionals embrace what they consider the only true and correct treatment regimens. These usually entail the distribution and use of standard drugs or "narcotics" produced by huge pharmaceutical companies, an overall industry nicknamed "Big Pharma."

The world's largest and richest drug companies have stabbed their proverbial hooks deep into the processes that run the American Medical Association and the federal Food and Drug Administration, also known as the FDA. Do you think these giant organizations truly care more about eliminating your pain and disease, or for making big bucks for themselves and for their shareholders?

Well, from my perspective, greed plays an overriding and predominant role in the development of the various strategies and policies of these organizations. Most standard physicians follow and embrace this often-ineffective medical routine and they dislike the fact that I'm willing to stand tall and openly proclaim this fact. Ultimately, the big loser is you, the consumer, average patients who usually are given no other option than to consume unnecessary and potentially addictive drugs, at least in some cases.

Yes, now is the time for you to dig deeper into the underlying causes of pain, and to discover the various standard treatments that are likely to cause potentially harmful complications or unnecessary addictions. Just as important, you can look toward the path that I show, filled with natural remedies and treatments. Many of these strategies are specifically designed to target pain, in many cases eliminating such symptoms altogether.

Chapter 7

Embrace and Benefit from the Tremendous Power of Prayer

Each day while alone in my office, and on Sundays at church services, I quietly pray for the physical recovery of my patients and for their individual improvements against the ravages of pain.

Like millions of other Americans, I strongly believe in the awesome power of prayer. According to an article in "USA Today," a whopping 83 percent of people responding to a survey said they believe that God answers our prayers. And, just as impressive, 92 percent of those surveyed indicate they believe there is a God.

According to the Pew Research Center's Forum on Religion and Public Life, a 2007 survey indicated that six out of 10 Americans reported that they pray every day.

The same U.S. Religious Landscape Survey indicated differences in the frequency of prayer, the amount of such activities conducted by people from various religions, and the income, age and gender of the faithful. Among the survey's findings:

- Age groups: A total 68 percent of people older than age 65 pray every day. That's the highest percentage of any age group surveyed, according to a forum press release. The smallest percentage from any surveyed age group that prays daily is from ages 18-25 at 48 percent; the percentage totals steadily increase with each progressively older age group, before cresting at the age 65 and above bracket.

- Gender: Sixty-six percent of females pray daily, compared to only 49 percent of males

- Income levels: Sixty-four percent of lower-income individuals earning less than $30,000 yearly indicate they pray daily, compared to only 48 percent of people who earn more than $100,000.

Throughout my medical career, I have seen many cases that seemed to show that the power of prayer generates undeniably positive results that some people would consider "miracles." Many of these improvements in the various medical conditions of these individuals might have resulted from the power of the mind, specific medical treatments, or perhaps even instances of unexpected natural recovery.

As a physician, I concentrate on scientific- and natural-related treatments rather than serving as a spiritual or religious advisor. Nonetheless, to any patient who happens to ask, I give my honest belief that prayer can and does serve as a significant and powerful force.

Data Shows the Mega-Powerful Force of Prayer

During the past several hundred years, there have been numerous well-documented and verified cases of people who have been condemned to die—only to eventually survive the execution process, possibly thanks at least in part to the tremendous power of prayer.

As you can very well imagine, each of these surviving individuals endured intense physical and emotional pain during the execution process. But in each of these cases, including some that involved the awesome power of prayer, the condemned people survived and then were allowed to live.

One of the best-documented cases involved soldier Wenseslao Moguel, sentenced to face a firing squad on March 18, 1915, after being captured during the Mexican Revolution. Eight bullets ripped through Moguel's body during the standard phase of the execution. Immediately afterward, an officer fired a bullet through this condemned man's head at close range in order to ensure the job was done.

Yet Moguel later escaped after managing to survive, apparently able to "play possum" and act like he was dead immediately after the execution process despite his intense pain. Twenty-two years later in 1937, Moguel appeared on the "Ripley's Believe It or Not" radio show, while photographers captured gripping images of his ravaged face and body.

Among some of the other cases verified by various historical documents and news reports, along with the accounts of various witnesses:

- John Henry George Lee: Sentenced in England to hang for the axe bludgeoning death of a woman, on Feb. 23, 1885, he stood at the gallows waiting for the trap door to fall beneath him—but a release malfunctioned on the device. Executioners attempted a repair, but the trap door failed a second time.

Frustrated personnel worked to effect repairs a third time, but it failed once again. Amid the confusion, guards returned Lee to his cell, and upon hearing of the incident an official reduced the sentence to life imprisonment. Twenty-two years later in 1907 officials reviewed Lee's case and then released him from prison.

- William Duell: In 1740, officials in the village of Tyburn, London, hanged Duell at age 16 along with four others for the rape and murder of a girl. Later that day, a servant noticed that Duell was breathing after the body had been stripped naked and laid on a board at a surgeon's hall—where the corpse had been brought to be anatomized. Two hours later this "dead man" was able to sit up in a chair, and upon hearing of his recovery officials commuted his death sentence.

- Anne Greene: In about 1630 at age 22 in England authorities hanged Greene after wrongly accusing the woman of killing a child whom she actually had given birth to as a stillborn. Some historians believe that Greene had conceived the child when seduced by a grandson of her employer. During the execution, she was pushed off a high ladder, and witnesses reported they let her body dangle from the rope for about a half hour. The body was then taken to a doctor for use in anatomy lectures. Yet doctors who converged for the dissection heard the body take a breath. Greene then spoke a few words after being revived. Upon hearing of her survival, an official reprieved the execution sentence. Green then lived another 15 years, during which she married and had three children.

- Joseph Samuel: In 1801, hundreds of people gathered in Sydney, Australia, to watch the hanging of this man who proclaimed his innocence despite his murder conviction. Authorities scheduled him to die along with another condemned man. After Samuel prayed, a cart on which he and the other condemned man had been standing was driven away. But the rope snapped from around Samuel's neck. Executioners then tied Samuel to a second rope and then dropped him again. But the second rope slipped and his legs touched the ground. Upon hearing these details, the governor considered the events as a "sign from God" and then commuted the sentence to life in prison.

- Willie Francis: In 1946, a Louisiana jury convicted this African-American of murder after his defense lawyer failed to offer any defense whatsoever. On May 3, 1946, executioners strapped Francis into an electric chair and flipped the "on" switch. According to various witness accounts and news reports, as electricity cascaded through his body, the teenager started screaming "Take it off! Let me breathe!" Another report indicated that Francis had proclaimed, "I'm not dying." In a subsequent investigation, authorities concluded that an intoxicated prison guard had improperly set up the portable execution chair. During the subsequent year the Supreme Court rejected Francis' appeals that officials had violated his Fifth, Eighth and 14th Amendment rights. Later, after he apparently had sufficient time to "make peace with God," Francis was then successfully executed on May 9, 1947, one year and six days after the unsuccessful attempt.

These compelling and magnetic true-life tales of survival epitomize equally gripping stories that now occur every day. Without any publicity whatsoever, patients suffering from usually fatal levels of illness and extreme pain survive, literally beating the odds. At emergency rooms, patient rooms and in doctor's offices nationwide, some patients get the much-awaited joyous news that their diseases have gone into remission and their pain subsides. The vast majority of these occurrences get little or no publicity.

Indeed, miracles are occurring every day, seemingly all around us and yet we rarely ever realize all this is happening. Those of us within the medical profession who serve as close insiders to individual cases take great pride when such instances occur.

Unlike most condemned people who know they will die after a last-possible appeal gets denied, for many standard patients there is almost always at least some degree of hope—for as long as they remain alive, and for as long as they feel the pain.

Certainly, those of us in the medical profession who deal with daily life-and-death decisions often notice that this longtime saying remains true—"Man can live about 40 days without food, about three days without water, about eight minutes without air, but only for one minute without hope."

Some Survivors of Intense Pain Far Surpass Mere Hope

Going well past the point of what many of us would consider mere "miracles," some people have "free-fallen" inside planes that literally plummeted to earth from many miles up in the sky—and lived to tell about their experiences. These are not cooked-up or phony tales by any stretch of the imagination, but actual occurrences that epitomize the great possibilities for hope.

As a prime example, on Jan. 26, 1972, media outlets worldwide flashed the news that stewardess Vesna Vulović had survived a 33,000-foot drop after explosives brought down a Jat Aircraft in the former Czechoslovakia, now the Czech Republic. Journalists reported that Vulović lapsed into a 27-day coma while physicians worked to repair her broken skull and three broken vertebra.

After Vulović awakened, the news media quoted her as saying "the man who found me says I was very lucky. He was in the German Army as a medic in World War II. He knew how to treat me at the site of the accident."

Needless to say, this incident involved intense pain, while also serving as another significant reminder to us all that survival and the eventual eradication of pain remain possible for those who envision the best-possible outcomes.

"At such moments you realize that you and the other are, in fact, one," said Joseph Campbell, a 20th Century American mythologist, writer and lecturer. "It's a big realization. Survival is the second law of life. The first is that we all are one."

Chapter 8

Some People Need to Suffer Extreme Pain to Survive

As uncomfortable as this might sound, the sad truth remains that nature or physical conditions sometimes force us to endure extreme pain in order to survive.

A legendary example of this gained international acclaim in the case of American mountain climber Aron Ralston, 27 years old when left with no choice other than to use a crude knife to amputate his own arm in 2003 when a boulder trapped the limb.

A widely acclaimed 2010 movie about Ralston's ordeal, "127 Hours" starring James Franco in the title role, featured intense, extremely graphic scenes of the amputation. The depiction was so realistic that many people fainted dead-away when watching in theaters.

Remember, physical pain sometimes afflicts more than merely its victims, but also individuals forced to watch others as they suffer. Conversely, many of those who personally observe other people suffering pain sometimes feel intense, gratifying emotional pleasure.

Ralston's gripping story exemplifies the unstoppable force of the human spirit, especially those willing to suffer intense pain in order to survive. The hiker had disappeared after failing to tell anyone of his plans for the Utah excursion. Once trapped, he spent a five-day period slowly drinking what little water he had. As those supplies dwindled, Ralston scratched his name and the supposed date of his impending death on the canyon wall. While the limb remained trapped, he also filmed a "goodbye video" for his relatives.

Still more than 15 miles from his truck after freeing himself, while bleeding profusely Ralston had no choice other than to rappel more than 30 yards down a sheer canyon wall. Then, while walking out of the canyon under a hot midday sun he came upon a couple from the Netherlands hiking with their son. These good Samaritans on vacation contacted the authorities and gave him water.

Gradually this excruciatingly painful ordeal resulted in many benefits for Ralston, who regularly made appearances on all major late night talk shows. The "New York Times" reported that by his mid-30s and boosted with celebrity status, Ralston commanded $25,000 per speaking engagement and no less than $37,000 for such international appearances. Boosting Ralston's star power, "GQ" made him 2003 Man of the Year, and "Vanity Fair" hailed him as "Person of the Year" for that period.

Yes, as an overall society, Americans love winners, champions in the battle against severe pain, and we often put them on proverbial pedestals, dead-center in the media spotlight for all of us to admire and adore. If Ralston had died alone from exposure when lost in the wilderness, most people would never have known he existed.

The character of General George Patton as portrayed by George C. Scott in the hit 1972 movie "Patton" made this "winner-gets-admiration" philosophy clear while addressing troops and standing in front of a wall-size American flag—proclaiming that "Americans traditionally love to fight. All real Americans traditionally love the sting of battle."

This memorable scene played a significant role for Scott's acting career, especially after his Patton character went on to observe that "Americans love a winner and will not tolerate a loser. Americans play to win all the time, and we don't give a hoot in hell for a man who lost and laughed."

I Watched the Ravages of Pain Caused by War

While growing up in the American Midwest in the late 1930s through most of the 1940s, and later in California in the 1950s, like other kids and young adults my age I occasionally visited theaters to watch typical cowboy movies and war films. In most battle scenes primary characters died heroically, many giving extensive heart-felt speeches until taking their final breaths. Most times the good triumphed over the evil.

All those sugary perceptions got shot out of my mind in 1969, as I served as a chief pathologist and medical team officer, while witnessing some of the worst, bloodiest battles of the Vietnam War. After some battles, I personally had the duty of conducting autopsies one-by-one on hundreds of my slain comrades. Some of these essential tasks forced me to work in a small building, the room crammed high with stacked caskets each holding one of our slain soldiers. Extensive nose-clogging stench filled the room, partly because some bodies had begun the decay process. Many corpses had been immersed in muddy marshlands and were bloated with gas gangrene.

Complete Pain

My assigned duties required that I work with great diligence and efficiency, while avoiding any inkling of becoming overly emotional. The exploded and bullet-riddled insides of their bodies exposed me to the horrors that intense physical pain can impose on a human being.

Yes, the real General Patton in the previous great American war talked about the winners. From Patton's view, this seemed to apply to those of us capable of pulverizing our battlefield enemies before victoriously returning home in good health perhaps to revel in admiration at celebration parades.

But the eye-tearing scenes in the autopsy room, coupled with my crews' necessary deployments and their efforts to attend to our wounded comrades taught me a big lesson—that those who suffer extreme pain and die deserve honors as heroes, too.

Just as important, for me on a personal level, I used these many incidents as my own personal call to arms in learning, growing intellectually and eventually striving to provide the best medical services possible to my many civilian patients. From that point forward, more than ever before, I dedicated my professional life to the eradication of pain and disease. All of us deserve to pursue the perceived goals of happiness, especially thanks to the ultimate sacrifices made by these brave soldiers.

"Heroism is not only in the man but in the occasion," said Calvin Coolidge, the 30th President of the United States from 1923-1929.

Chapter 9

The Lack of Pain Adds to the Mysteries Facing Researchers

A s if the basic physical properties involving physical pain weren't already enough to amaze and confound researchers, there also are rare cases of people who fail to feel any such sensations whatsoever.

Referred to by physicians as "congenital insensitivity to pain" or "congenital analgesia," an extremely small percentage of people suffer from the inability to suffer physical pain, a phenomena that impacts a barely detectable segment of society. Unproven and undocumented comments hint that this affliction often hails among certain people from homogeneous societies—regions where most individuals are essentially similar to each other as an overall group.

Some scientists believe that for any species or segment of its population to thrive and remain as a vibrant, successful life form from generation to generation at least some biodiversity remains essential. In essence, biodiversity recognizes the differences between separate individuals of the same species within a specified ecosystem. Such factors, in turn, help ensure that a specific species within the ecosystem will remain healthy or able to adapt effectively to potentially adverse conditions.

And, adding to the mystery, researchers also conclude that some instances of congenital insensitivity to pain might be hereditary, passed from parents to their children. Progressive illnesses such as Hansen's Disease—commonly known as "leprosy"—can progressively destroy the nerves. Thereafter, scientists fear, the parents could possibly pass the illness to their offspring.

While serving as a primary and necessary essence of life, physical pain fails us when such sensations disappear and thereby become unable to do their job of signaling problems. Paradoxically, the permanent lack of such sensations becomes just as tragic as feeling physical pain. Each occurrence expresses a great potential problem. They are:

- Feeling Pain: The sensations of too much physical pain can gradually or suddenly bring about painful emotional situations as well, sometimes robbing people of the will to live or stealing away any hope of recovery.

- Lacking Any Pain: Countless diseases or potential injuries might erupt while the individual and his necessary immune system response mode fail in duties to react to illness and wounds. This, in turn, might prevent the nerves from sending to the brain critical information about pain in order for the person to generate adequate or necessary responses for healing. Thus, the complete and permanent lack of pain persists.

"Few tragedies can be more extensive than the stunting of life," said Stephen Jay Gould, an American paleontologist and evolutionary biologist in the late 20th Century. "Few injustices deeper than the denial of an opportunity to strive or even to hope, by a limit imposed from without—but falsely identified as lying within."

Meet a Person Who Never Feels Physical Pain

In 2005, "People Magazine" reported the compelling story of Ashlyn Blocker, who at age 5 suffered from congenital insensitivity to pain. Among the child's various pain-inducing behaviors reported by the magazine:

- Head: Slammed her head against the walls, shrugging at the site of blood on her face.

- Hand: Left her hand in the muffler of a gas-powered mower.

- Fingers: Put her precious little fingers into a door frame, before the device crushed them.

- Ants: Failed to notice when hundreds of ants started biting her, instead telling relatives that she couldn't get the dirt off her skin.

- Mouth: Badly bit her own lips, cheeks, and tongue, "causing so much damage that she began knocking out her front teeth."

As reported by "People," Ashley's parents Tara and John had to strike a delicate balance between striving to ensure the child's safety, while also offering her "a normal childhood." The child caused so much damage to her hands, the magazine said, that her parents had to wrap them in athletic tape.

"She looks like a little boxer," her mother told the magazine. "We don't want Ashlyn to live in a bubble. We've learned what to worry about and what not to worry about, and we give her space."

The lack of any pain and discomfort is so potentially harmful to the human body that Ashlyn faced the risk of overheating during the day. As a result, teachers at her school always ensured that the child had a water bottle on her desk.

At the time of this initial story, Ashlyn had recently suffered from tonsillitis that had gone undetected for six months. Her family and medical professionals were striving to teach her how to detect signs of potential infections such as appendicitis.

Following this extensive education process, Ashlyn learned to find her mother whenever she saw blood, and to ask if food was cool enough to eat, "People" said. All along, the girl still managed to feel some physical sensations such as hugs and kissing.

"She's got the best laugh in the world," Tara said, adding that "I would give anything, absolutely anything, for Ashlyn to feel pain."

Extensive and Ongoing Studies Remain Necessary

In studying the various vital differences between the sensation of pain and the lack of it, medical professionals potentially can make great strides in studying and quantifying the effects of dreaded diseases such a Hansen's Disease—commonly called leprosy.

Contrary to legend, the limbs and various appendages of people with leprosy never fall off as the disease progresses. Yet as a result of infection those areas of the body can become diseased or numbed. Leprosy can cause extensive damage to the peripheral nerves vital in sending pain signals to the brain, while also damaging mucus and the upper respiratory tract.

Leprosy remains mysterious, largely because symptoms often exhibit themselves suddenly. Some of the afflicted live normal lives without realizing they have the disease because the leprosy is in an incubation period of three to five years—and sometimes extending up to 30 years.

On the positive side, according to at least some reports, 95 percent of people are immune to the potential ravages of leprosy. And when people are eventually diagnosed, after just a few weeks of treatments they no longer can transmit the disease.

Another common misconception apparently involves a mistaken belief that the disease has been wiped out worldwide. In 2007, the BBC reported that during the previous 20 years, 15 million people worldwide had contracted the disease.

The urgent need for continued study of leprosy stems largely from the ravages and eventual death this disease often inflicts on much or all of the nervous system. By devising effective and essential methods of stopping this disease's progression, perhaps scientists can also develop superior pain treatment methods.

Chapter 10

The Human Genome Project
Offers Tremendous Hope

Although science still lacks a significant, comprehensive "cure-all" for pain, researchers assisted by physicians and medical experts have made tremendous progress in recent decades.

Much of this success stems from the Human Genome Project, in which scientists have mapped all 20,000-25,000 genes in our bodies. The bulk of this initial work occurred from 1987 to 2003, when scientists announced that they had chronicled or recorded all basic gene structures that operate the body's physical and functional systems.

For many generations to come, medical professionals and physicians will likely use this vital information in developing essential treatments and drugs for a wide variety of specific conditions. Pain likely will become a prime target of these efforts.

According to various medical journals and news reports, experts reviewing and studying the project's massive database already have determined that hereditary genetics often play a role in passing the tendency for pain to subsequent generations. Just as compelling, some individuals apparently have a predisposition to certain types of pain.

Adding even more questions to the complex mysteries of the human body, researchers also report that they have found that some individuals also inherit an inclination for inflammation and perhaps even tendencies for excessive or chronic pain.

These general findings come as no surprise to medical historians who point out that in 1866 the monk Gregor Mendel discovered that common peas displayed characteristics of inherited traits. Along with James D. Watson, in the 20th Century a British biologist and neurologist, Francis Crick used Mendel's research as the basis for their own Nobel Prize-winning discovery that the double helix of genes forms a primary basis of life.

The term "double helix" is used in molecular biology to describe double-stranded molecules that form DNA—scientifically called Deoxyribonucleic acid—a nucleic acid that contains genetic instructions for the basis of life. The double helix phenomenon also plays a significant role in RNA—Ribonucleic acid—a macromolecule deemed necessary in order for all known forms of life to exist.

Through much of the 20th Century, scientists used the findings of Watson and Crick as the basis for significant discoveries in a wide variety of crippling or fatal diseases. These painful maladies include breast cancer, cystic fibrosis, Down's syndrome, and many other debilitating conditions.

Buoyed by these numerous medical advances, scientists are working to delve much deeper into individual paired chromosomes in order to determine how to eliminate pain. In order to do this with any effectiveness, at least from my personal view, researchers will need to continue their ongoing and relentless efforts to methodically review and analyze each building block of the entire Human Genome Structure.

Look For Significant Progress Every Day

Without letup, researchers that you probably never heard about are keeping busy going step-by-step in methodically reviewing and analyzing each of the four primary building compounds of life—largely in an effort to identify and essentially wipe out the ravages of physical pain. These basic compounds are:

- Adenine: Serving as a chemical component of both DNA and RNA, adenine plays a variety of significant roles including cellular respiration, essential metabolic reactions and processes within cells in order to convert nutrients into energy.

- Guanine: Derived from purine, an organic compound, guanine plays a critical role in the formation of the double-bonded ring systems of both DNA and RNA.

- Cytosine: In the base pairing bond discovered by Watson and Crick, cytosine serves as the basis in the formation of guanine's three hydrogen bonds.

- Thymine: Scientists say this plays a critical role in stabilizing nucleic acid, a basic and necessary part of both DNA and RNA.

Following the rules or requirements of the human genome structure as mandated by Mother Nature, these four purine-based building blocks form a wide array of complex sequences. These, in turn, form an integral series of codes, building blocks for the master plan that makes each person unique and functional—plus how we feel and react to pain.

The Key Triggers of Pain Will be Tricky to Find and Isolate

For scientists and physicians seeking to eradicate physical pain, the key to success hinges largely on identifying specific points that trigger the signals of such symptoms. Among these, the most essential characteristics are commonly called SNPs, referred to by physicians as "single nucleotide polymorphisms." This factor remains highly critical, primarily because SNPs can produce subtle variations in the manner in which separate individuals respond to specific illnesses, injuries or various forms of trauma.

Besides regulating or signaling varying responses to pain, the SNP system and process also plays a significant dual role in determining, regulating and managing how our cells respond, absorb and react to drugs, food and essential nutrients such as vitamins.

Needless to say, as a result of these highly complex and interdependent processes, physicians and medical professionals are now faced with a formidable task. The key to success hinges on creating medical strategies to effectively balance these various factors, essentially an integral and difficult-to-achieve balancing act.

"Being on a tightrope is living, everything else is waiting," said Karl Wallenda, the famed founder of the popular Flying Wallendas daredevil circus act of the 20th Century. Wallenda died in 1978 at age 73 when he fell from a tightrope 121 feet above ground between two towers in San Juan, Puerto Rico.

Yes, in a sense, while working diligently to generate effective pain remedies, researchers of the human genome structure are essentially walking a tightrope. But unlike the sturdy and predictable ropes or wires that Wallenda walked, the subtle variations within the gene map of the human body can unexpectedly sway or move in unpredictable ways.

Herein rests the key to success, continually refining and fine-tuning our potential abilities to manage or isolate gene structures that regulate everything from swelling, stress, inflammation, detoxification and a vast array of other bodily functions.

Despite these many formidable challenges, scientists should proceed with enthusiasm and careful due diligence in actively pursuing these hoped-for solutions. After all, as the late movie star James Dean once said, "Dream as if you'll live forever, live as if you'll die today."

Discover Your Unique DNA Characteristics

With continued progress, individual consumers hopefully will someday be able to receive a comprehensive analysis of their own personal, individual gene structures.

On a comprehensive level, this would enable a person to determine his or her own propensity toward swelling, specific types of pain, abilities to detoxify, limit inflammation, and a wide array of other necessary bodily functions.

As the old saying promises, "knowledge is power." But even more important from the perspective of those eager to reduce pain, the ability to get an individualized DNA map could open up doors leading to significant physical recovery. Such intricate discoveries might tend to infuriate huge pharmaceutical companies that profit from the propensity of consumers taking ineffective drugs or who undergo unhelpful treatment regimens.

Every significant "advance in natural knowledge has involved the absolute rejection of authority," said Henry Thomas Huxley, a 19th Century English biologist known as "Darwin's Bulldog" for advocating Charles Darwin's theory of evolution.

When the time comes for each of us to acquire our personalized DNA maps in a private, accurate manner, we all should eagerly seek this essential information. Particularly those of us suffering from extensive physical pain should be able to look to such data as a guide or roadmap on how we can best manage our personal lifestyle behaviors. The gene map has already become critical for chemo-sensitivity testing of cancer patients.

For instance, a person who discovers from his personalized DNA map that he has a propensity to suffer from excessive swelling in certain joints, could modify his exercise routine in order to prevent or alleviate the probability of suffering such pain. Depending on the specific afflictions identified, potential ways to prevent or lessen pain could range from the consumption or avoidance of certain foods to the active exercise of certain muscle groups.

Chapter 11

Survive and Thrive Despite Physical Pain

"It is not the strongest of the species that survives, nor the most intelligent that survives," said Charles Darwin, a 19th Century English naturalist who wrote the controversial "On the Origin of Species" featuring his theory of evolution. "It is the one that is the most adaptable to change."

Sharing the same birthday, Feb. 12, 1809, as the 16th President of the United States, Abraham Lincoln, Darwin died in 1882 at age 73. Darwin's theories of evolution and survival failed to protect him from the ravages of severe illness and various physical sicknesses beginning at age 29 in 1838.

Yes, due to the very nature of pain and its unbendable predictability, even the world's greatest, most famous geniuses have failed to escape horrible aches and illnesses. To this day, many historians remain confounded and perplexed, unable to cite the exact cause of the precise illness that began bothering Darwin in his late 20s.

While some historians hint that Darwin's illness may have been at least partly psychosomatic, others note that he suffered progressive weakness, nausea, headaches, horrible bouts of vomiting and even illnesses that limited his work to two hours daily.

Until subsequent advances in medicine dictate otherwise, countless people today still suffer from difficult-to-diagnose illnesses and mysterious pains that are hard to treat.

"Every age, every culture, every custom and tradition has its own character, its own weaknesses and its own strengths, its beauties and its cruelties," said Herman Hess, a German-born Swiss novelist, poet and painter of the late 19th and early 20th Centuries. "It accepts certain sufferings as matters of course, put up patiently with certain evils. Human life is reduced to real suffering, to hell, only when two ages, two cultures and religions overlap."

Certainly Darwin's theories on evolution ignited intense international controversy, often instigating the ire of Christians who insisted the first human beings were Adam and Eve—created by God as described in the Holy Bible's Book of Genesis. Darwin's writings gave a different view, stating that modern humans gradually evolved from other animals.

Today, as physicians and medical professionals strive to develop and implement the best-possible, non-addictive painkillers, the longtime issue of creation often takes a back seat to the overriding necessity of "pure science." And while some religious beliefs shun or prohibit the use of modern medical techniques, modern doctors understandably find themselves ignoring the issue in order to concentrate on remedies to treat illness and pain.

"It is not clear that intelligence has any long-term survival value," said Stephen Hawking, an internationally acclaimed theoretical physicist and cosmologist who suffers from neuromuscular dystrophy, a medical condition related to amyotrophic lateral sclerosis—which degenerates the body's vital central nervous system.

Use the Best Medicines and Treatments Available

While physicians dutifully strive to improve and modify methods of controlling and managing pain, people worldwide struggle daily to find effective, affordable relief from such sensations. The vast majority of these heartbreaking cases go unnoticed, including cases where pain leaves some individuals bedridden for years or even decades.

Even the world's wealthiest, most famous people often struggle to find the best possible methods and the most skillful physicians to manage their relentless, life-altering pain.

Often seeking to hide their physical afflictions from the public, some celebrities have used their giant financial resources to scour the world in hopes of benefiting from adequate pain relief. Details of these struggles often hit the front pages of supermarket tabloids, getting far more publicity than common everyday consumers could hope for.

Born in 1946, the widely respected actor, screenwriter and filmmaker Sylvester Stallone of "Rocky" and "Rambo" movie fame, was so frustrated by persistent knee pain that he finally resorted to holistic Indian methods to relieve the discomfort, according to news media reports.

Generating just as much widespread publicity pop star Paula Abdul, a former judge on the hit TV show "American Idol," reportedly has suffered from an extremely serious medical condition—complex regional pain syndrome, a chronic and progressive disease.

Journalists have reported that Abdul suffers from chronic pain and earaches from this condition, apparently triggered in 1979 at age 17 when she was injured in a cheerleading accident.

In 1980 at age 23, future movie star Melanie Griffith, famous for such films as "Working Girl," was hit by a car while walking across Sunset Boulevard in Los Angeles. According to various news reports, the mishap lead to a lifetime of physical and emotional distress, her severe hip and neck injuries leading to narcotic-drug addictions.

In recent decades, numerous other top-name celebrities have traveled to my West Coast clinic seeking relief from pain and illness. While news of their maladies hit front pages of publications such as the "Los Angeles Times," in most cases journalists never learned that certain famous individuals benefited from my clinic's various treatments.

Like all physicians, I strive to protect the privacy of my patients, giving both celebrities and everyday citizens my full and undivided attention in administering medical care.

"Even the smallest victory is never to be taken for granted," said Audre Geraldine Lorde, a 20th Century Caribbean writer, activist and poet. "Each victory must be applauded."

Chapter 12

Psychosomatic Situations Complicate the Field of Pain

Complicating the overall study, diagnosis and treatment of standard pain, many people also suffer from what physicians refer to as "psychosomatic behavior." The Miriam-Webster Dictionary defines this condition as matters involving, related to or concerned with "bodily symptoms caused by a mental or emotional disturbance."

In many cases involving psychosomatic symptoms of pain, physicians often cite emotional or physical stress as a primary instigating factor. Intertwining this mix, chronic physical stress also can lead to general or "actual" illness.

First off, lay people and medical professionals need to remain cognizant that an individual sometimes suffers stress in situations where he or she feels a complete or near-total lack of ability to control unpleasant events. Major potential stressors could include everything from an inability to generate a sufficient income to worries about a lover's potential infidelity or earning adequate grades in school in order to graduate.

Sadly, at least in my personal opinion, many people tend to place unwarranted blame on those who experience psychosomatic medical conditions. Anyone who would call such a patient "nuts" or "loony" should seriously consider withholding such thoughts. After all, as a result of their perceived conditions, psychosomatics sometimes suffer emotionally, spiritually and financially while also experiencing potentially debilitating physical symptoms.

Even so, some of the world's most respected behavioral experts still insist on placing blame on psychosomatics for bringing about their own medical conditions. As a result, this complex and often poorly understood issue will likely remain a hot topic, even as new and much-wanted medical advances gradually evolve.

"Lose-win people bury a lot of feelings. And unexpressed feelings come forth later in uglier ways," said Stephen R. Covey, author of the bestseller "The Seven Habits of Highly Effective People." "Psychosomatic illnesses often are the reincarnation of cumulative resentment, deep disappointment and disillusionment repressed by the win-lose mentality."

Whether or not we agree with such assessments physicians need to treat such conditions with just as much care and concern as any other serious medical condition.

Aggressive Medical Treatments Can Help Psychosomatics

Within the extensive overall practice of behavioral medicine, the detection and effective treatment of psychosomatic behavior can depend on variations of a wide range of specialties. These can include—but are not necessarily limited to—everything from psychiatry, physiology, and allergies to dermatology and many more areas of medicine.

Psychosomatics often complain of specific or vague pains, some described as severe or mild and rather vague. After at least a short time in practice, just about every new doctor has heard a patient describe a small or vast array of perceived physical complaints that lack any underlying standard, general medical basis.

More than merely a figment of the psychosomatic patient's imagination, these perceived ailments including the perceptions of pain are very "real" in their minds. In fact, the force of the mind is so powerful that some psychosomatics experience or express observable symptoms such as rashes, convulsions or body temperature changes.

"You have power over your mind, not outside events," said Marcus Aurelius, a Roman emperor in the second century after Christ. "Realize this, and you will find strength."

Embracing a similar strategy, in formulating and implementing treatments for psychosomatics, many physicians and medical professionals focus on the use of positive thinking or even what some lay people refer to as "mind over matter."

This is not to imply in any way whatsoever that physicians strive to employ treatments that delve into the paranormal. Instead, many treatment experts emphasize the spiritual realm of the personal belief system generated within the mind, which some people believe holds just as much great power as the body.

Psychiatrists and General Practice Physicians are Making Great Strides

With headquarters in Bethesda, Maryland, the Academy of Psychosomatic Medicine has helped take a significant leadership role in dealing with such conditions.

The Academy's published mission states that it represents psychiatrists "dedicated to the advancement of medical science, education and healthcare for persons with co-morbid psychiatric and general medical conditions, and provides national and international leadership in the furtherance of these goals."

Available online at its Website, apm.org, the Academy distributes or provides subscriptions to its journal entitled "Psychosomatics." Updated publications contain in-depth articles on issues that the organization's members consider pivotal or urgent advancements in research and treatments for such people. A vast array of topics or research reports include studies or treatments involving anxiety, AIDS, malignant melanomas, Parkinson's Disease, and many other serious, painful medical conditions.

Physicians treating specific patients for "verified" or diagnosed conditions sometimes hear those individuals complain of perceived pains or other psychosomatic symptoms that apparently were not caused by the diseases or wounds. Such instances obviously might tend to complicate attempts to achieve the best possible treatments for the primary underlying illness.

Such conditions have been so integral to the overall practice of medicine that the "Psychosomatics" publication has been produced and disturbed for more than 160 years. Annual meetings of medical professionals involved with or interested in these respected journals draw many of the world's most dedicated physicians who specialize in such diagnosis and treatments.

"Leadership is based on inspiration, not domination; on cooperation, not intimidation," said William Arthur Ward, a 20th Century inspirational writer.

Psychosomatic Medicine Has a Vibrant, Important History

Historians tell us that physicians have known about psychosomatics since at least the 10th Century, when two psychologists and physicians first noted these conditions during the medieval Islamic period. Through their studies, research and medical practices, Ahmed ibn Sahl al-Balkhi and Haly Abbas determined that the psychology and physiology of a patient can impact each other.

According to a 2005 "International Medical Journal" article, these physicians noted correlations between people who are both mentally and physically ill, and those who are healthy. Then, during the 11th Century, a famed Persian physician and philosopher known today by the single name "Avicenna," recognized and described the significant impact that emotions can play on our bodies.

Significant advances occurred in the study and identification of psychosomatics throughout the 20th Century, particularly beginning in the early 1970s when many physicians started using the biosemiotic theory as a basis for such medicine. A German,

Thure von Uexküll, a scholar of psychosomatic medicine, and his colleagues, developed the biosemiotic theory that attempts to:

- Integrate: Melding the conclusions researchers have made in scientific biology and "semiotics," a term used to describe the studies of the symbols and signs from various cultures. In the view of John Locke, the 17th Century English philosopher, semiotics can relate to everything from words, to the nature of things, and their relationships with each other. In the 19th Century, American scientist, philosopher and mathematician Charles Sanders Peirce defined semiotics as signs used by "intelligence capable of learning by experience."

- Interpretation: This is the process where people assign meaning to the various signs, symbols and messages, often via verbal messages or by sight. Without necessarily knowing this is being done, a person sometimes uses his perceptions of logic or mathematical data to interpret information that arrives in the forms of signs or symbols.

- Paradigmatic shift: The blending of scientific biology and semiotics causes a "paradigmatic shift," a term used to describe changes in previously accepted basics that involve the theory of science.

Essentially, from the view of scientists, this complex integration and interaction of the basic science of biology with the system of signs or messages can effect a person's perception of life. According to some published reports, this forms "the theoretical basis for psychosomatic medicine."

Jakob Johann von Uexküll, a Baltic German biologist in the late 1800s and early 1900s, used the "unwelt" theory that people and other animals can generate or interpret different meanings from certain signs or communications—although they share a similar environment. This "unwelt" concept also is often considered to play a significant role in the approach that today's physicians, psychiatrists and medical professionals take when dealing with the psychosomatic phenomenon.

The Psychosomatic Condition Causes Many Physical Disorders

Physicians report that people experiencing psychosomatic medical conditions often suffer from physical diseases, stemming from life's everyday stresses. Psychiatry has made recent advances in determining which mental factors—if any—were the likely cause of a specific individual's psychosomatic-related medical problem.

The wide array of documented medical conditions include Irritable Bowel Syndrome, chronic fatigue syndrome, peptic ulcers, lower back pain, bacterial infections, and high blood pressure. Some of these maladies can emerge as serious and sometimes life-threatening medical conditions.

All along, scientists and medical professions stress the importance of avoiding any use of the incorrect term "psychosomatic illness," when referring to certain types of mental illnesses or "somatoform disorders." Individuals experiencing the mental illness of somatoform disorders sometimes exhibit physical symptoms similar to those conditions experienced by people who have been in accidents or who have certain illnesses.

In summary, the basic differences between these overall conditions are:

- Somatoform disorders: This is a disorder that can result from various mental factors. Such patients often become unnecessarily worried or stressed when physicians are unable to diagnose a specific cause, a determination necessary to describe a pain or an ailment.

- Psychosomatic medicine: This is a field of medicine that involves various medical specialties, hinged largely on the bodily processes and on the health of people. Personal behaviors, social conditions and psychology are among factors that play key roles. As a subspecialty of psychiatry and neurology, this condition also can sometimes benefit from positive thinking or what physicians sometimes call "the power of suggestion."

Ultimately, as with any serious medical condition, patients should never attempt to diagnose themselves, particularly in matters that involve real or perceived pain. Only a certified and licensed medical professional can make an accurate diagnosis, before recommending and implementing treatments or prescriptions.

Severe, Intense, and Crippling Pain Can Erupt

Worsening matters from the perspective of patients, the various conditions involving psychosomatic medicine and somatoform disorders can result in what lay people and physicians sometimes refer to as a "pain disorder." Such conditions can become so severe that a patient sometimes becomes disabled, preventing him or her from common everyday activities.

As with most severe medical conditions, those suffering from intense pain should visit a physician or medical professional as soon as possible. Early diagnosis and treatment could possibly go a long way toward stopping or preventing the progression of symptoms. According to some researchers, the onset of any pain disorder can hit both genders at any age.

Taking on a so-called "life of its own," some instances of pain disorder reportedly stem from an actual injury or illness. Thereafter, following the point when the underlying or primary medical condition is otherwise "cured," the patient continues to perceive severe pain or discomfort—when in fact there is no underlying medical basis for such symptoms.

Indeed, the accurate diagnosis of "real" or "perceived" pain is an extremely complex and integral process that sometimes involves extensive medical testing over an extended period of time. In today's complex world, medical professionals from a wide array of specialties find themselves faced with formidable challenges in accurately pinpointing and treating painful conditions that stem from psychosomatic medicine and somatoform disorders. Thus, both patients and physicians share the vital responsibility of remaining vigilant in sharing and exchanging such information in order to bring about effective results.

"Learning is the beginning of wealth, learning is the beginning of health," said Jim Rohn, a 20th Century American entrepreneur, motivational speaker and author. "Searching and learning is where the miracle process all begins."

Chapter 13

Self-Mutilation Inflicts
Serious Pain

While most people struggle to fight pain and go to great means to eliminate such sensations, every day worldwide many individuals intentionally inflict severe wounds on themselves. The vast majority of these people are average little-known citizens, while some of those who harm themselves are widely acclaimed celebrities and movie stars.

Among the most notable was actor Johnny Depp, star of many blockbuster films including "Pirates of the Caribbean," "Edward Scissorhands," "Sleepy Hollow," and "Fear and Loathing in Las Vegas." According to various media reports, Depp self-inflicted eight scars on his upper left forearm while a young man.

"Talk Magazine" has quoted Depp as saying in an interview that there was no ceremony when he inflicted these wounds—"It wasn't like 'Okay, this just happened. I have to go hack a piece of my flesh off." And, in 1993 "Details Magazine" also quoted Depp on the issue: "My body is like a journal in a way. It's like what sailors used to do."

The mysterious or at least mystifying occasions when people physically harm themselves this way apparently happens more often than many of us realize. And intentionally inflicting pain on ourselves occurs in many forms, sometimes referred to as "self-harm," "deliberate self-harm," "self-injury" and even "self-poisoning." These occurrences serve as prime examples of how the instinctive need to avoid—and even to experience—physical pain plays an instrumental role in the human psyche. Among other instances:

- Angelina Jolie: An Academy Award® winner and the star of numerous films, born in 1975, Jolie inflicted wounds on herself while in her early teens, according to a 2001 issue of "Rolling Stone Magazine." Media reports say that in a 1999 TV interview Jolie admitted that by harming herself, "I was trying to feel something."

- Courtney Michelle Love: Born in 1964, this rock 'n' roll musician and actress, was once quoted by "Spin Magazine" as admitting to having run around naked and cutting her own arms—"I think self-destruction is given a really bad rap. I think self-destructiveness can also mean self-reflection, can mean poetic sensibility, it can mean empathy, it can mean a hedonism and a liberationism and a lack of judgment."

- Diana, Princess of Wales: This late 20th Century former member of the British Royal Family, who died at age 36 in 1997 of injuries suffered in a Paris car crash, had revealed in a 1995 TV interview with the BBC that she was a self-injurer who cut her own legs and arms. Diana admitted that "you have so much pain inside yourself that you try and hurt yourself on the outside because you want help."

The mere notion of why someone would actually injure and inflict pain on themselves might seem highly perplexing, especially to anyone trying to eliminate severe sensations such as those caused by certain cancers or injuries from car crashes. After all, from the perception of most societies and religions, the human body is a sacred temple, essentially a precious gift from God that should never be harmed.

"How strange is the lot of us mortals," Einstein said. "Each of us here for a brief sojourn, for what purpose he knows not, though he senses it."

Some People Injure Themselves for a Blood Rush

Movie star Christina Ricci once admitted to "Spin Magazine" that she had occasionally used cigarettes to burn her own arms. From this, she told the publication, "You get this endorphin rush. You can actually faint from pain, it takes a second, a little sting, and then it's like you really don't feel anything. It's calming actually."

While such statements might boggle the minds of many people, medical researchers and some physicians report they're making great strides in determining reasons for such seemingly perplexing behaviors.

People who intentionally injure and cause physical pain to themselves choose a variety of methods, but cutting seems to reign as the most frequent method. Other common methods include hitting or banging body parts, scratching—and even intentionally interfering with the natural wound-healing process. Among the variety of compelling factors or conclusions reached by medical researchers:

- Suicide: Apparently most cases of self-harm are not considered life-threatening, at least according to a 2007 article in "Psychoanalytic Psychology." And while some researchers caution against any tendency to categorize self-harmers as suicidal, at least by some accounts there may be an increased risk of suicide among such individuals.

- Similar behaviors: Although substance abuse and certain eating disorders can cause physical damage, such activities should not be listed as instances of self-harm, according to a 2007 article in the "Journal of Clinical Psychology."

- Frequency: Instances of self-harm are not considered frequent, but have been occurring in greater frequency since the early 1980s, according to a 1997 publication, "Stuart and Sundeen's mental health nursing, principles and practice."

- Age groups: The greatest percentages of people who suffer from episodes of self-harm are adolescents and young adults from ages 12-24, according to an article in a 2005 edition of the "Journal of Youth and Adolescence." All age groups are affected, including those in advanced maturity.

- Personality traits: Researchers consider self-harm as a symptom of a condition that physicians call "borderline personality disorder," according to the "Diagnostic and Statistical Manual of Mental Disorders." Doctors describe such disorders as prolonged instances where an individual's personality function is disturbed. Symptoms of such disorders can include an inability to logically differentiate between life's choices, and instability in maintaining moods. People suffering from such disorders also sometimes experience instability or chaotic episodes in their behaviors, self-identity, and relationships.

- Terminology: Some people take offense to any use of the term "self-inflicted injury" or "self-mutilation," descriptions occasionally viewed as either worrisome or inaccurate. All along, the phrase "self-inflicted wounds" refers to soldiers who intentionally harm themselves in an effort to get dismissed from battlefield duties. In addition, researchers describe instances where prison inmates intentionally harm themselves, apparently in attempts to get removed from potentially harmful situations.

Ultimately, at least from my view, pinpointing and treating each individual's reasons for self-harm often requires extensive analysis and review by mental health professionals—and in some cases, in conjunction with consultations with standard or Homeopathic physicians as well.

"Sometimes I lie awake at night and ask, 'Where have I gone wrong,'" said Charles Schulz, a 20th Century cartoonist, creator of the popular "Peanuts" comic strip. "Then, a voice comes to me, 'This is going to take more than one night.'"

Review an Extensive List of Potential Causes

Besides borderline personality disorder, scientists point to a vast array of other potential triggers that can possibly ignite instances of self-harm. These conditions range from schizophrenia and substance abuse to depression and anxiety.

As if all these many complex and life-alerting conditions weren't already enough, some analysts and physicians also must consider a wide array of other potential lifestyle or life-altering situations that are sometimes associated with self-harm. According to various published reports, these range from substance abuse and sexual abuse to instances where an individual is emotionally abused by other people.

"Out of intense complexities, intense complexities emerge," said Winston Churchill, the 20th Century prime minister of Great Britain.

Meantime, some observers insist that instances of self-harm might result from an attempt to grab the attention of other people, while others describe such theories as inaccurate. Lots of people who inflict self-harm upon themselves strive to hide those scars, either self-conscious or feeling guilty about their behaviors.

Some self-harm suffers have opened up, speaking publicly about how suffering such pain impacted them emotionally. Irish-born movie actor Colin Farrell, star of such films as "Phone Booth," "Minority Report," and "Tigerland," admitted in an interview with "GQ" magazine that he loved the sensation of pulling out or yanking at his hair while in his early teens. "Yeah, before it's left the follicle, right—that moment right before it's left. And, then the … I just … love it." Medically, this is termed "trichotillomania."

According to a 2004 book by Jessica Kingsley, "Deliberate Self-Harm in Adolescence," physicians and the medical industry lack a system of diagnostic criteria to establish and identify instances of self-harm. A 1994 book, "Self-harm, perspectives from personal experience," indicates that many people who harm themselves would like physicians to develop such a standard. To address this concern, in 2010 officials announced that the upcoming fifth edition of the "Diagnostic and Statistical Manual of Mental Disorders" would list instances of non-suicidal self-injury as the criteria for such a conclusion.

Genetics Sometimes Plays a Role in Self-Harm

Scientists tell us that an extremely rare inherited or genetic disorder, Lesch-Nyhan Syndrome results from an enzyme deficiency. This condition causes body fluids to amass an excessively high amount of uric acid. Sometimes the disorder results in symptoms associated with mild retardation, gout or kidney problems, and inadequate muscle control. Some of the worst symptoms first start erupting in the second or third year of life, when people suffering from this syndrome begin harming themselves—causing extreme pain.

These behaviors sometimes involve biting the lips, tongue or fingers. And the vast majority of these cases, an estimated 85 percent of them, involve boys. Eventually in some cases as the disorder progresses some youngsters start violently banging their heads against hard objects.

Based on various research reports, medical professionals sometimes misdiagnose or misinterpret instances of the disorder, wrongly characterizing or diagnosing symptoms as being the result of mental conditions that spark instances of self-injury.

For individuals with this syndrome, some medical professionals deem self-harming behaviors as uncontrollable. Meantime, the syndrome's sufferers experience cognitive impairments, which physicians sometimes have difficulty identifying—possibly due to the patients' behavioral problems. According to some published reports, caregivers might become frustrated or angry when sufferers of the syndrome refuse snacks or react to displays of kindness with cold, rage-filled behaviors that sometimes include spitting or involuntary swearing.

Some researchers have concluded that there is no way to effectively treat the disease's behavioral aspects. The "deep-brain stimulation" treatment, which resulted in a decrease of certain self-harming behaviors, was discussed in a "New Yorker" magazine article written by Richard Preston, published in August 2007. The treatment involves the surgical implantation of a brain pacemaker that sends electrical signals to tissue.

Brain pacemakers have been used in treating a variety of physical conditions including chronic pain, epilepsy, Parkinson's disease and clinical depression, according to a variety of published reports, including a 2007 article in "Nature Reviews Neuroscience."

Other symptoms of this illness are often treated with standard procedures used in handling each specific condition, such as specified medicines for gout, excessive uric acid, and kidney stones.

Self-Harm Produces Emotional Reactions

After intentionally harming themselves, some people report that they feel a sense of calm, almost as if they're relieved and have a new-found sense of control. And as unbelievable as this might sound, lots of them also describe a new-found or rediscovered sense of feeling "real," almost as if they're finally alive or somehow able to function.

Marie Chapain, an award-winning American writer and Christian counselor has been quoted as saying—not specifically while referring to instances of self-harm—that a "lack of discipline leads to frustration and self-loathing."

Whether such observations dig deep into the fabric of self-harming behaviors remains to be seen. Many people who intentionally harm themselves report that experiencing physical pain serves as a desired distraction from their personal emotional pains, according to Helen Spandler's 1996 publication, "Who's Hurting Who? Young people, self-harm and suicide."

Even as such observations persist, however, medical professionals seem to remain inconclusive on precisely how to treat painful self-harming behaviors, according to a 1998 article in the "British Medical Journal." Despite such conclusions, in my personal and professional opinion, as the years progress researchers, mental health experts and general physicians will continue significant studies into this condition—while developing new or refined attempts at solutions and treatments.

Chapter 14

Discover the Complexities of Münchausen Syndrome

The realm of intense human pain and suffering takes on a macabre and horrific mode in cases where parents hurt children. Scientists have documented cases where mothers intentionally inflict pain and severe injury on their children in order to generate attention or sympathy. Beginning in the 1950s, such instances began receiving the label "Münchausen Syndrome By Proxy."

The vast majority of perpetrators are mothers, reportedly up to 90 percent of cases, according to a 2006 article in "Forensic Science International." Researchers cite instances where the parent inflicts actual harm or extreme pain on the child, while some cases involve fabricating and describing bogus or phony symptoms to medical professionals.

Münchausen Syndrome gained widespread attention in 1977, when a professor of paediatrics at the University of Leeds in England, Roy Meadow, chronicled behaviors of two mothers involved in separate cases of child abuse. Meadow described a case where a mother used excessive amounts of salt to poison her child, and an instance where a woman used her own blood when tampering with her toddler's urine sample.

Meadow's findings generated controversy in the 1990s when he testified in criminal trials that news media reports say resulted in wrongful convictions of murder. In 2006, "The Times" in London published an article stating that after being freshly knighted as "Sir Roy," Meadow was "plunged into disgrace" by the controversy.

In 1993, Meadow testified in the criminal case of Beverly Allitt, subsequently convicted of injuring nine children and killing four, and given 13 sentences of life in prison. The "Times" reported that Meadow's reputation then reached a new high, going on to testify in many criminal trials—some involving deaths previously described as involving instances of natural sudden infant death syndrome. News reports quoted him as saying that there was no evidence that such instances commonly referred to in England as "cot deaths" run in families, while "child abuse does." This became commonly known as Meadow's Law, that "one cot death is tragic, two is suspicious and three is murder."

Controversy Erupted

Prosecutors in England convicted at least 80 women whose children might have suffered from Sudden Infant Death Syndrome through the 1990s of murder, manslaughter or infanticide on the basis of Meadow's Law, the "Times" said. Meantime, Meadow's professional prestige blossomed, and largely in recognition of his work on behalf of the health of children, he was knighted in 1998.

However, according to various news media accounts, the professor's standing in the medical community took a substantial downturn as a result of a trial the following year. Prosecutors accused lawyer Sally Clark of killing her sons Christopher and Harry, who died at ages

14 weeks and eight weeks respectively. While Clark proclaimed her innocence, pediatricians gave diverse views on her possible guilt.

Proclaiming his certainty that the deaths involved murder, while addressing the jury Meadow "testified that the odds against two cot deaths in the same family were 73 million to 1," the "Times" said. "He calculated the figure by squaring the 8,500-1 odds of cot death in a normal family. It was as likely, he said, as an 80-1 horse winning four consecutive Grand Nationals. This sensational and insensitive analogy was to become a suicide note to his career."

The court sentenced Clark to life in prison after her conviction, after the woman had wept openly proclaiming "I could not believe something like this could happen twice." In 2000 the judges denied her appeal that claimed Meadow's data was misleading, and also stating that families experiencing an initial cot death are more likely to suffer a second. Two years later the court overturned the convictions after medical tests indicated that a bacterial infection likely caused at least one of the deaths.

"Professor Meadow suffered a second blow when called to give evidence in the case of Trupti Patel, a pharmacist accused of killing her three children in 2003," the "Times" said. "After a high-profile trial, in which the Professor's statistical evidence was torn to shreds by the defense, jurors found her not guilty within 90 minutes. The Solicitor General, Harriet Harman, effectively banned him from court work."

This development opened the proverbial floodgates for lawyers who represented many of the women who had been jailed at least partially based on what some people considered as Meadow's questionable math. Many defense lawyers filed appeals. Within the following year, a court freed one of the women, Angela Cannings, convicted for killing two of her children.

England's General Medical Council then launched an investigation, and Meadow eventually underwent what the "Times" described as three weeks of relentless questioning during the probe—which resulted in officials pulling the then-retired professor's license to practice. The newspaper reported that his testimony was denounced as "naive, grossly misleading, incompetent and careless."

Meadow appealed and in 2006 the London High Court upheld his defense, deeming his punishment as disproportionate. One justice proclaimed, the "Times" said, that Meadow was guilty of nothing more than a simple, honest mistake.

Such Cases Become Extremely Complex

Any discussion or review of the complexities of physical pain should involve the emotional and psychological motivations of people who inflict such sensations on others. Along with self-harm, the issues of Münchausen Syndrome by Proxy and Doctor Meadow play an integral role in our overall understanding of such medical conditions.

Simply stated, general physicians, psychiatrists and behavioral experts face difficult social issues and integral medical decisions when handling such cases that involve pain and intentionally inflicted injuries.

Only by carefully reviewing and treating each instance—while also developing accurate statistical procedures—can doctors make significant advances in rendering and developing such treatments. In this combined effort, physicians, patients and government authorities must remain continually vigilant in identifying and addressing the vast array of specific symptoms. While the overall phenomenon of Münchausen Syndrome by Proxy often involves intense controversy, this condition remains a "real" and very serious matter.

All along, the general mainstream news media needs to work to uphold a higher standard when reporting such instances. For instance, journalists generally reported Meadow's findings of 73 million-to-1 odds as statements of fact, rather than delving into specifics of how and why this doctor generated his analysis.

Following the various court rulings, some women convicted of killings largely on the basis of Meadow's testimony stated that they had yet to hear an apology from him. And in 2004, according to some published reports, Meadow's ex-wife, Gillian Paterson, was quoted as implying that she considered him a misogynist—a person who hates women.

Long before these issues erupted, the Roman emperor from the second century after Christ, Marcus Aurelius, seemed to hit the target of such analysis and societal conflicts dead-center when he observed that, "Think of this doctrine, that reasoning beings were created for one another's sake; that to be a patient is a branch of justice, and that men sin without intending it."

Münchausen Syndrome by Proxy Involves Serious Consequences

Parents suspected of inflicting Münchausen-style abuse or death upon their children face serious consequences across the United States. Various laws and governmental policies in most states require medical professionals to report suspected cases to authorities.

And physicians treating young patients also must take reasonable measures to prevent suspected or potential abusers from inflicting any additional harm on children. In Judith A. Libow's 1993 book, "Hurting for Love: Münchausen by Proxy Syndrome," a wide array of potential warning signs are mentioned. These range from noticing puzzling cases where treatments fail to follow their usual course, to instances where parents seem unusually fascinated by hospital gossip or seem highly knowledgeable of medical details.

Just as distressing, as Libow reports, some parents who secretly inflict such harm on their children become highly demanding of physicians and medical staffers, always ordering more opinions or tests. Doctors also cite incidences where mothers display an unusual degree of calmness, sometimes even though the child suffers serious medical problems. Another potential telltale sign involves extensive family histories of unexplained medical conditions.

Keeping these urgent issues in mind, doctors and especially emergency room personnel or physicians at clinics need to remain vigilant in watching out for such cases.

"Few things are impossible to diligence and skill," said Samuel Johnson, an 18th Century British author and essayist. "Great works are performed not by strength, but perseverance."

Chapter 15

Would You Literally Walk on Fire?

Throughout recorded history in numerous societies, many people have literally walked on fire as if to prove that the power of their minds can prevent or ignore excruciating pain.

Commonly referred to as "firewalkers," such people sometimes walk barefoot across extremely hot coals, stones or embers. Most of the time these people somehow manage to avoid displaying or experiencing any sign of discomfort or injury.

In a sense, such instances involve people who attempt to convey a distinct message to the world around them, essentially saying: "I'm powerful. My mind is everything, and the possibility of any pain at all means virtually nothing to me."

Some cultures use these occasions to test an individual's faith. Sure enough, within the psyche of humans, any perceived or actual victory over pain is often viewed as a great achievement worthy of eternal praise and of much well-deserved adulation.

Many religious faiths and diverse cultures have practiced this longstanding custom. Eastern Orthodox Christians, Taoists, Buddhists, and practitioners of certain African faiths have engaged in firewalking for thousands of years.

While any reasonable physician would never suggest or even recommend such behavior, firewalkers and people who advocate such activities refer to the process as healthy or at least inspiring good health and personal growth. Some firewalkers strive to strengthen or at least train their minds to focus on positive outcomes.

"A man is but a product of his thoughts, what he thinks he becomes," said Mohandas Gandhi, a pre-eminent advocate of civil rights and an ideological leader in the culture of India in the late 19th Century and early 20th Century.

Firewalkers Have Permeated Many Cultures

Historians tell us that firewalkers have thrived and engaged regularly in "walking on fire" since at least 1,200 years before Christ.

People interested in the study, elimination and management of physical pain can easily find themselves mesmerized and intrigued by the many tales and historical accounts of such behavior. To most of us living in today's Western world, the mere notion of such a stroll can literally send shivers down our spines and make goosebumps erupt from head to toe.

"Love is a fire," said Joan Crawford, a 20th Century American movie actress. "But whether it is going to warm your heart or burn down your house, you can never tell."

Indeed, there is little denying that almost anyone who tries to walk on fire for the first time needs to employ what lay people often call a "leap of faith." Such attitudes might seem reasonable, because after all, since early childhood just about all of us are either taught to avoid extreme pain or we learn the hard way as toddlers, positioning ourselves to rarely ever repeat the same mistakes. Any small child who inadvertently puts his finger on a hot stove almost always learns to avoid repeating such behavior.

Besides expressions of religious or spiritual faith, some cultures use fire walking as an integral part of initiation processes, or even—as amazing as this might sound—as a form of spiritual or mental healing. The practice grew increasingly popular in the 1970s when advocates of "positive thinking" began embracing this process as a way for their students or practitioners to cross an essential "right of passage."

Primary figures in this social transition across the American cultural landscape included Tolly Burkan, widely praised by his advocates as the founder of the Twain Harte, California-based "Firewalking Institute of Research and Education."

Avoid Any Attempt to Walk on Fire without Experts

Attempts to "walk on fire" atop coals, blazing-hot rocks or other burning materials sometimes results in extensive injury, especially to anyone making such a stroll without expert guidance. Truly, in their effort to show their own strength of "mind over matter," some people go too far, too fast without first attempting to get sufficient information.

When performed correctly, scientists say, pre-planned and well-choreographed fire walking efforts result in little or no injury whatsoever. Experts give much of the credit to the natural abilities of chosen materials to conduct or absorb the heat, rather than sending blazing hot temperatures outward into or through the walker's skin.

As a result, when performed properly the burned materials lack the essential heat capacity necessary to inflict injury. In addition, in a process called "thermal effucivity," the natural variations in heat levels within the embers or coals and the feet are different, scientifically decreasing the likelihood that high temperatures can successfully transfer into the body.

As Einstein eloquently stated, "everything is theoretically impossible, until it is done."

Even so, unforeseen, unplanned for or unwanted factors sometimes emerge, thereby occasionally interfering or changing the results of otherwise predictable outcomes. Such unwanted factors have resulted in overly enthusiastic firewalkers suffering burned feet when they remained atop the flaming areas too long, eliminating any chance of benefiting from the conductivity of burned materials. Other unfortunate individuals become too excited and even run atop coals, thereby forcing their feet deep into dangerous portions of the extremely hot embers.

As if all these problems weren't already enough to cause extensive worries, some careless participants leave unintended foreign objects on the standard burning materials—thereby igniting unnecessary and extremely dangerous flames. Adding to this danger, anyone who attempts to walk on flames with previously wet feet poses the risk of getting hot materials stuck to the body—potentially causing extensive injury.

Chapter 16

Human Sacrifice Enters the Realm of Pain and Physical Suffering

Throughout history, various religious beliefs have motivated or inspired some people to seriously injure or even kill each other. Herein the instinctive human nature of avoiding or inflicting physical pain sometimes gets intermixed with the emotional, spiritual, mental or theoretical belief systems of people from many cultures.

In some societies and religious rites, ceremonial events involved the slaughter of animals or human beings. Some belief systems mandated or inspired the slayings or bodily punishments as perceived ways of appeasing or pleasing the Gods. While many of us in today's modern cultures would view such behaviors as ruthless and unnecessarily cruel nonsense, to those who participated the carnage seemed forgivable and even required.

"All outward forms of religion are almost useless, and are the causes of endless strife," said Helen Beatrix Potter, a late 19th Century and early 20th Century English conservationist, author, and illustrator. "Believe there is a great power scientifically working all things for good, believe yourself and never mind the rest."

Engulfed in their own religious dogma and eager to believe the spiritual beliefs taught to them, people in many cultures for the past several millennia have slain, carved up, tortured or mutilated other human beings. In almost every instance, the goal of inflicting intense pain, extreme suffering and ultimately death emerged as a primary objective.

The vast array of participating cultures ranged from tribal societies, headhunters and even religious systems that involved cannibalism— the wretched act of killing or even cooking human beings in order to eat them. In some cases this happened as if the flesh of any person were a much-south-after delicacy.

Pain Reigns as the Very Nature of Mankind

Sadly, the inflicting of pain and the avoidance of such sensations remains prevalent in almost every aspect of the human condition. In fact, pain or the effort to avoid experiencing it hails as a primary factor in why we buy or avoid purchasing from a vast and seemingly endless array of products and services available in everyday modern life.

We might avoid buying a car, fearful of the emotional pain incurred by the responsibility of making payments—coupled with the perceived physical pain that we could potentially suffer, while laboring hard in order to secure the necessary finances. Conversely, we might choose to buy the same vehicle, fearful that any lack of such transportation could result in a perception that we're weak or inadequate—thereby making us perceived as potentially weak or at least vulnerable to painful injury.

The essence of pain delves within the core of our natural human bodies, while crossing into many aspects of our personal spiritual realms or individual belief systems. Human beings have intrinsically known or at least sensed this integral, interlinking system of pain-motivating sensations—seemingly since the beginning of most recorded religions or spiritual beliefs, and even within some systems of political dogma.

For instance, the basic foundation of Buddhism, the bedrock of that belief system explains the Four Noble Truths—starts with the proclamation that suffering hails as a universal aspect of the physical experience of the human existence. Like many religions or spiritual belief systems, Buddhism never advocates or encourages the senseless or random infliction of human pain and suffering. Even so, violence and the infliction of extreme pain have still permeated many belief systems and cultures.

Leo Tolstoy, the great Russian novelist of the 19th Century and early 20th Century, told us that "we have become so accustomed to the religious lie that surrounds us that we do not notice the atrocity, stupidity and cruelty with which the teachings of the Christian church is permeated."

Many Religions Embraced Pain and Intense Suffering

A vast majority of us God-fearing, peace-loving Christians throughout today's modern society—myself included—point out that 21st Century advocates of our faith understandably become repulsed by the very notion of physically hurting or inflicting pain on anyone in the name of religion.

Yet our current philosophies and good-intentioned behavioral strategies fail to erase the fact that physical pain and death have reigned as integral to our belief system and to those of many other currently respected religions for thousands of years.

In fact, the very essence of our great faith and belief acknowledges that our Lord and Savior Jesus Christ suffered intense physical pains, during his final torture and eventual crucifixion as an atonement for the sins of all human beings. And since that historical juncture just more than 2,000 years ago, those who have embraced Christianity have exacted horrific amounts of pain, suffering and downright cruelty on other people in the name of religion.

Without question, the very essence of physical pain permeates all of our lives, even as we embrace various belief systems in an effort to relieve suffering, especially in instances where the natural death process enters its final phases. Various forms of "the death rite" or the "final sacrament" remain sacred, essential cores of numerous religions.

This seems natural to almost anyone who cherishes a love-based, deep-rooted spiritual or religious belief. These philanthropic and caring motivations strike me as natural and inspiring reactions, since from the human perspective—at least when seen through the eyes of many religions or spiritual belief systems—the devil himself represents pain of many types.

James W. Forsythe, M.D., H.M.D.

The Devil Reflects the Image of Pain

Virtually every significant culture, religion and spiritual faith throughout history has recognized "the devil," usually characterized as the complete opposite of good—an enemy of all people, of our souls, of our bodies, and of God as well.

And, although physical pain is "good" at least in the sense that it warns us about current or potential physical problems, such sensations are generally considered as wretched and even wicked. These are similar qualities often attributed to religious figures considered the equivalent of the devil, known by such names as Lucifer, Satan or the Dark Angel.

While many faiths perceive the devil as an extremely powerful or even supernatural entity, the very essence and perception of physical pain from the human perspective often carries similar connotations. On an equally strong level mentally, physically and spiritually, the devil is known to rob people of their good-intended free will, stealing away personal wisdom and hampering attempts at enlightenment. Similarly, physical pain can and does rob people of their abilities to make wise decisions, to think or behave in a clear, level-headed, selfless and keenly focused manner.

Just as disturbing, at least from the perspective of many God-fearing, caring and loving Christians, physical pain and even mental anguish sometimes results in sinful or selfish behavior—in essence reflecting the base, vile and lower nature of interaction among individuals.

"We are each our own devil, and we make this world our hell," said Oscar Wilde, the Irish writer and poet from the late 19th Century.

Indeed, just as almost all of us within the human race strive to avoid, prevent and eliminate physical pain, we also need to refuse such sensations to allow us to dwell on or to carry out negative behaviors—potentially harmful to ourselves and to others. All of us, collectively and individually, should help ourselves and each other to overcome temptations to allow pain to point our hearts and our minds in a negative direction.

"I often laugh at Satan, and there is nothing that makes him so angry as when I attack him to his face, and tell him that through God I am more than a match for him," said Martin Luther, the 15th and 16th Century priest who founded the Protestant Reformation.

Pain Motivates Much of the Human Spirit

Often in the name of religions or spiritual belief, the willingness of people to inflict intense physical pain on others has put a wretched mark on much of human history. The many instances of human sacrifice have crisscrossed ancient Egypt and Mesopotamia, to the early Neolithic and Greco-Roman cultures of Europe—impacting the Germanic and Slavic societies as well.

Strangely similar and often heartlessly cruel ceremonies and ritual slayings also originated in ancient China, Tibet and India plus vastly different regions across the Pacific Ocean. Archaeologists have chronicled countless instances of human sacrifice across the Pre-Colombian Americas and Mesoamerica, where leaders of some cities inflicted severe pain upon and killed many of their own citizens as a perceived method of attempting to resolve disputes.

As recently as a few thousand years ago, some people in the Mayan cultures of Central America hurled human beings down giant sinkholes in the earth in hopes of pleasing water gods. And just more than 500 years ago, the Aztec culture in an area now known as Mexico City sacrificed tens of thousands of people.

Instances of horrifically painful human sacrifice also occurred in South America in the pre-historical Bronze Age of 3,000 years before Christ, and reportedly less than a few hundred years ago within some native tribe cultures of North America

The countless methods of inflicting extreme injury or eventual death, depending on specific cultures and eras, have ranged from poison to stabbings, beheadings, and even extremely slow executions designed to generate the most intense, prolonged pains possible.

Thankfully, specific instances of human sacrifice are extremely rare and almost non-existent in today's world. We can look at this as a sign that perhaps to a great degree most societies have collectively become "more civilized." Even so, war and extreme violence remain prevalent on a daily basis, as evidenced in daily reports in the general news media. Perhaps this stems in part from the fact that human beings instinctively know that physical pain and death shall always remain.

Controversial Research Shows People Voluntarily Torture or Kill Others

A social psychology experiment conducted more than 50 years ago still ignites controversy, concluding that people often willingly follow orders of their superiors who command that they inflict pain on other individuals.

Complete Pain

The "Milgram experiment" first performed by a Yale University psychologist in 1961 indicated that a vast majority of people will obey an authority figure—even in instances when such commands conflict with the subservient person's conscience and values.

In the experiment, people who volunteered as "teachers" communicated via speaker phones with their "learners" in separate rooms while unable to see each other. Every time a student gave an incorrect response to a pre-designated question, the teachers were to flip a switch administering an electric shock to the learner. And every time the learner gave a wrong answer, the shock level was increased by 15 volts.

Unbeknownst to these teachers, however, their learners or students were actors who never actually received or suffered from the shocks. These actors, technically called "confederates," played pre-recorded sounds upon receiving each increased degree of shocks.

Much of the time, the teachers nervously laughed or behaved in a stressful manner when shock levels reached a dangerously high 135-volt level. At that point, many teachers told their "experimenters" who moderated these sessions that they did not want to continue. And, to heighten the sense of pain and suffering, the unseen actors or confederates began banging on the wall in the separate but adjoining room.

Whenever teachers indicated that they no longer wanted to continue, the experimenters assured these instructors that they would not have to face responsibility for their actions. According to various published reports, when the teachers expressed a desire to stop the sessions the experimenters gave pre-determined comments such as "please continue," the "experiment requires that you continue," or "it is absolutely essential that you continue."

The experimenters halted the sessions in instances where the teachers still wished to stop after four consecutive verbal prods. And, when a teacher applied three consecutive 450-volt shocks to an individual student, experimenters ended a session.

Shockingly, to pardon the pun, a whopping 65 percent or just a fraction under a full two-thirds of participants designated as teachers administered the maximum 450 volts at least once. Each participant who inflicted these maximum-level shocks had paused at least briefly, questioning whether to continue.

Are People Inherently Cruel in Matters of Pain?

In 1974, just 13 years after this initial research, the professor, Stanley Milgram, wrote an article stating that although the teachers' ears were ringing with the screams of their victims, "authority won more often than not." While these results might strike some of us as disturbing or perhaps even inaccurate, numerous similar or nearly identical studies have reached fairly identical conclusions or results at other universities since then.

From the perspective of many people, findings such as these might indicate at least partly why or how human beings have been willing to obey the destructive commands of their leaders throughout much of history. These include the countless instances of human sacrifice in many cultures, and also amid the Holocaust in which Nazis killed millions of Jewish people immediately before and during World War II.

By some accounts, the Milgram experiment is still considered so important that the original equipment including an event recorder and simulated shock generator are kept at the Archives of the History of American Psychology at the University of Akron in Ohio.

Although some psychologists have questioned the ethics and the conclusions of these studies, there is little denying that human beings are capable of inflicting devilish levels of pain on other people.

On the positive side, everyone from political leaders to medical professionals and top psychologists continues to work diligently in pinpointing and addressing such "flaws" in the human psyche. Hopefully over time our youngsters from many cultures can be taught beginning at an early age to question authority—especially in instances where a culture or society's leaders insist upon the use of excessive pain-causing or lethal force.

Some People Embrace the Wicked Philosophies or Actions of Others

Adding to the mystique of why people often willingly inflict pain on others, additional studies and research have indicated that lots of us "conform" or embrace the behaviors of individuals from within our own cultures.

According to results from the Asch conformity experiments first conducted in the 1950s, people are more likely to conform, emulate or imitate the behaviors or beliefs of others when at least three or more individuals behave a certain way in the same group.

By some accounts, even a small minority of dissidents from a culture can have an impact on whether an individual conforms to a specific way of thinking or behaving.

The world around us "is made up for the most part of morons and natural tyrants, sure of themselves, strong in their own opinions, never doubting anything," said Clarance Darrow, a civil libertarian heralded as a country lawyer in the early 1900s—famous in part for defending thrill killers Nathan Leopold Jr., and Richard Albert Loeb.

With equally disturbing conclusions, in a study hailed as the "Hofing hospital experiment" in 1966 when ordered to do so by a physician, a whopping 21 out of 22 nurses obeyed the orders of a physician who told them to give patients dangerous doses of a drug. Thankfully, those who conducted this research used a placebo.

In the Hofing experiment, the nurses received phone calls from a physician that they had never met. During these conversations, the "doctor" ordered the nurses to administer dangerously high levels of a specified drug to certain patients, also telling these medical professionals that he would later sign for the medication.

Beforehand, those who conducted this experiment had placed a bottle of the fictitious drug in a cabinet—and in each instance the substance was not on a list of pre-approved medications. Some observers have argued that these nurses allowed themselves to be deceived, largely because of their own high opinions of the medical profession's overall standards.

Some People Generate Excuses for Inflicting Pain

Those of us interested in the detection and treatment of pain—both in its physical and mental forms—realize that some people who intentionally inflict such sensations on others strive to rationalize such evil-minded, selfish and senseless behaviors.

"It's the victim's fault that this happened," or this "pain does not matter because the person is less than human," such instigators seem to tell themselves. Some experts in social psychology often refer to such instances as "moral disengagement." Essentially instances like these sometimes involve the use of certain morals or values, in developing an excuse for inflicting pain or even death on other individuals.

For instance, the excessive or extreme torture of a terrorist might become justified and considered necessary when arguing that such action is "for the greater good." Taking this a step further, some instigators place the blame for these actions on their superiors who issued orders. And a juror who voted "yes" for an execution might blame "the jury," spreading the blame to others rather than accepting his or her own involvement.

"Cruelty is part of nature, at least part of human nature, but it is the one thing that seems unnatural to us," said Robinson Jeffers, a 20th Century American poet.

In order to inflict pain, some instigators strive to dehumanize their intended victims, thinking of these individuals as less than people as if the targets are "subhuman." Even more disturbing, at least from the view of those of us who abhor cruelty, much of society tends to blame victims of many kinds, from people who suffered injuries in accidents to those wounded in crimes.

When these factors come to play, lots of people within a particular society hold victims responsible for their own distress and difficulties, rather than placing the blame on those who caused the wounds or hardships.

Chapter 17
Seasoned Medical Professionals Fight to Win Against Pain

As acts of terrorism, war and common everyday metropolitan-style violence erupts daily worldwide, medical professionals, researchers and physicians are working feverishly to develop a wide array of new and effective cures for violence-inflicted pain and injury.

Mirroring a trend that has prevailed relentlessly throughout history, military experts and police professionals are continually seeking and implementing methods of preventing or lessening the likelihood of violence. Meantime, partly in an effort to address public demand of medical advancements necessary to address such violence-inflicted wounds, scientists and physicians are constantly devising ways to eliminate such pain.

In essence, as a profession and as a culture, we in the American society and within the international medical industry have found ourselves wrapped up in the never-ending cycle of violence. The very nature of the propensity of human beings to inflict pain on each other has forced or motivated physicians to develop new or highly skilled emergency room trauma strategies, and to work in the development of new or highly effective pharmaceuticals.

For those of us—especially people from the so-called "lay public"—learning about the many intricacies of pain for the first time, an essential educational process begins with the study of many integral and interlinked challenges and issues.

A key factor emerges involving matters related to why and how the medical industry has advanced and grown through the past several centuries, particularly in efforts to address physical pain.

Besides the never-ending quest to cure diseases, medical professionals from vastly diverse cultures have strived to eradicate physical pains that people intentionally inflict on each other.

People Have Used Pain to Achieve Their Selfish Desires

For thousands of years, human beings employed boundless creativity and ingenuity when devising horrific methods, systems and devices to inflict physical pain on one another.

Thankfully, only a handful of people seem to give such matters much thought these days. Yet for us to achieve any clear understanding of how physical pain damages our bodies, souls and psyches, we need to remain cognizant that humans are capable of horrific deeds— ranging from slowly boiling each other in oil to methodically and painstakingly cooking individuals in flames. In the Middle Ages, only the most experienced executioners were able to slowly cook the feet first, before methodically roasting the calves, thighs, crotches, torsos—all while keeping the screaming and wailing victim alive, before much-wanted death finally arrived.

Many of the most perverse torturers blinded their victims using sunlight, slowly castrated screaming individuals, or strangled them for as long as possible.

Besides ultimately causing death, a primary objective often remained the breaking of the human spirit in order to force a confession or a revelation of secret details.

Numerous societies have beaten or stoned the condemned as slowly as possible. As little as 500 years ago, some mid-European cultures strapped victims to wheels as thousands of cheering people watched executioners repeatedly slam huge hammers against the tied-up limbs of the condemned.

"Cruelty, like every other vice, requires no motive outside of itself—it only requires opportunity," said Mary Ann Evans, a 19th Century English journalist and novelist who wrote under the pen name George Eliot.

Mean-Spirited Tortures Prevailed for Centuries

Some cultures employed sadistic and wretchedly cruel tortures that resulted in intense physical pain without necessarily causing death. Some slave owners, revolutionaries or members of the aristocratic elite have used everything from pulling out fingernails to force-feeding victims until they bloated or even depriving them of sleep.

Some victims suffered horribly disfigured bodies, got their faces ripped to shreds so that they became difficult to look at, or suffered broken eardrums when forced to endure extremely loud sounds.

143

Battlefield tactics in some cultures have involved kneecapping, the intentional cracking or destruction of the knees usually by using a firearm as a battering ram.

A lengthy list of other torture methods ran the gambit of physical and psychological destruction, such as using hungry rats to slowly dig into the flesh or even sawing off limbs one by one while striving to keep the victim wide awake and alive for as long as possible.

Leo Tolstoy, the widely acclaimed Russian novelist and philosopher of the late 19th Century and early 20th Century, observed that "In order to get power and retain it, it is necessary to love power. But love of power is not connected with goodness, but with qualities that are the opposite of goodness—such as pride, cunning and cruelty."

Psychological Tortures Intensified the Problems

Creating and employing a vast array of devices for inflicting pain, some wicked, heartless and cruel despots have chosen to go far beyond once-common tactics such as tooth extractions, scalping, punching sensitive bodily areas, severe tickling or pouring hot tar and feathers on scantily clothed or naked victims.

The paraphernalia, tools or devices used to inflict severe physical pain has included electric shock instruments, or stretching wracks devised to slowly pull the body apart joint by joint.

Some unlucky prisoners in diverse societies in Europe and the early Americas were locked in stocks in public places, where everyday citizens often cruelly inflicted beatings or torture—compounded by suffering caused by exposure to the elements.

Especially in the 19th Century in some American cultures, police sometimes confined prisoners to physically painful "tramp chairs"— occasionally used to transport inmates or to restrain suspected or convicted criminals in communities too poor to build jails.

Herman Hesse, a Swiss novelist from the late 19th Century through the early 20th Century, pointed out that "every age, every culture, every custom and tradition has its own character, its own weakness and its own strength, its beauties and cruelties. It accepts certain sufferings as matters of course, puts up patiently with certain evils. Human life is reduced to real suffering, to hell, only when two ages, two cultures and religions overlap."

When Torturers Inflict Pain Deep Within the Psyche

Some political adversaries or enemies also experienced great personal enjoyment, perverse pride or even financial gain when inflicting various forms of psychological torture.

Perhaps the worst of these include mock executions, where victims are lead to believe they're about to get executed. But each time they're allowed to live without knowing beforehand of such a result. The cruelest practitioners of this method force victims to dig their own graves or to elicit what victims believe are their final statements.

The mind often seems to bend, crack or soften when the body is subjected to solitary confinement, deprived of all meaningful physical sensations such as light, the ability to see images or even to hear sound.

Adding horrific spice to this proverbial mix, some torturers intentionally administer highly addictive narcotics in hopes of permanently ruining their lives.

"My doctrine is this, that if we see cruelty or wrong that we have the power to stop, and do nothing, we make ourselves sharers in the guilt," said Anna Sewell, a 19th Century English novelist.

Some Experience Pleasure from Receiving or Inflicting Pain

Police, prosecutors, psychologists, psychiatrists and standard allopathic physicians occasionally face additional challenges in cases that involve people who enjoy receiving or inflicting pain.

Those who experience pleasure when inflicting pain on others engage in "sadism," while people that experience joy or sexual pleasure when receiving pain are involved in "masochism." Behavioral experts call the intermixing of sadism with masochism as "sadomasochism"—sometimes called "S&M."

Occasionally perplexed or even bewildered by these lifestyles, detectives, mental experts and medical professionals often strive to find answers or clues to what triggers such behaviors. Judging by the countless medical papers, research documents and news reports that I have seen through the years, depending on specific cases involved the experts cite everything from possible mental illness to potential strategies for avoiding stress.

The continued and consistent study of sadomasochism remains essential for the betterment of all society, especially because mind-boggling and harmful behaviors of this nature seem more prevalent than ever before.

Amazingly, however, many people also still insist that the overall practice of sadomasochism has benefits in incidents that never involve severe or permanent injuries. From this way of thinking, an individual can experience pleasure through the inflicting or receiving of pain in a manner that is not psychologically sexual in nature.

Amid this process, those who embrace or adhere to such lifestyles also point out the joy felt in experiencing pleasurable pain from strange or unexpected areas of the body.

Many People Become Offended Upon Learning of Such Practices

Naturally, some people find themselves repulsed and mentally anguished—internally pained—upon hearing about what they consider such strange and odd behaviors.

In fact, from the view of many people, the very act of inflicting pain upon other individuals in order to experience pleasure borders on sacrilegious. Indeed, many religious cultures and belief systems view the intentional infliction of pain as evil or devilish, contrary to the will and desires of the loving God who created us all.

Understandably, do to such perceptions, many sadomasochistic behaviors force prosecutors and even some medical professionals to come to grips with moral dilemmas. Chief among these confusing predicaments rests the question: "What are the boundaries of what all of us, individually and as a society, should consider 'right' or 'wrong?'"

147

For instance, some couples enjoy deliberately choking or strangling each other during sex, a process that sadomasochists and even some medical experts call "erotic asphyxiation." To at least some degree, this perceived pleasure stems from the temporary depravation of oxygen to the brain. If performed properly—at least from the perspective of some participants—the sudden and intense release of oxygen back into the brain once the strangulation stops causes an extraordinary, orgasmic sensation.

But when performed wrong, erotic asphyxiation can result in severe physical disability, irreversible brain damage, or even death. To be sure, no valid or reliable medical expert would or should ever condone or recommend such behavior. In fact, some physicians classify such behaviors as within the realm of mental disorders, due to the possibility that these actions will result in severe physical harm.

Some Participants Beg to be Choked

At an alarming rate, physicians and police find themselves forced to deal with the cases of people who literally pleaded to be choked almost to the point of death. According to some historical accounts, people from various cultures have engaged in this practice since at least the 17th Century.

Even today, as horrific and perplexing as this might sound, some people become so emotionally, physically or psychologically addicted to erotic asphyxiation that they beg or demand that their new or ongoing lovers choke them during sex.

Personally, I find such behaviors as disturbing and contrary to the basic norms of how civilized individuals should behave. Even so, no matter how we might individually feel about such matters, those of us in the medical industry or within the practice of psychiatry must continually work on treatments and solutions because that's our job, and because our profession demands that we strive to help others— while improving the quality of their overall health.

By their very nature, physicians hate or despise wars and other perplexingly harmful human behaviors. Even so, however we might feel personally about a particular issue, as medical professionals we still must respond to such occurrences to the best of our abilities.

An old Chinese proverb proclaims that "medicine can only cure curable disease, and then not always." Sure enough, those of us in the medical profession and people throughout all of society must realize that we all face perplexing dilemmas, morally, spiritually and physically.

According to a 1995 article in the "Journal of Forensic Sciences," an estimated 250 to 1,000 people die yearly when attempts at erotic asphyxiation go awry. Various news accounts and medical reports indicate that some of these victims died while attempting to experience such eroticism themselves without a partner.

Numerous deadly cases of erotic asphyxiation have sensationalized the news media during the past century. Some news reports have blamed the 2009 death of actor David Carradine in Thailand on accidental asphyxiation via the use of a rope, resulting in a case that some observers speculated might have involved eroticism.

Avoid the Deadly Choking Game

Like other physicians, I strongly urge people to avoid any attempts at erotic asphyxiation, no matter how enticing such prospects might seem to them. All along, another disturbing and potentially deadly behavior is sometimes called the "choking game"—also known as the "fainting game."

Not necessarily erotic or sexual, a choking game occurs when two or more people gather for the purpose of strangling each other to a point of near death in hopes of experiencing a sense of euphoria. To them, the temporary physical pain of being choked is well worth the perceived "high" of the eventual blood rush experienced when oxygen returns to the brain.

One of the primary or much-desired symptoms is hypocapnia, which occurs when the blood's levels of carbon dioxide become dangerously low. Besides the possibility of severe anxiety, this can cause numerous disturbing outcomes including blurred vision, and dizziness—or symptoms common from hyperventilation, such as muscle cramps or tetany, the involuntary contraction of muscles.

According to some published accounts including quotes from a London physician, Dr. Steve Field, fainting game behaviors differ from erotic asphyxiation in the sense that these actions are perceived as non-sexual, essentially a method to "get a high" without taking drugs.

Suggested or possible reasons for engaging in this perplexing behavior have ranged from wanting to feel intoxicated while avoiding the expense to peer pressure or even as a way for schoolmates to ditch class. While all this might sound enticing or potentially exciting to some people, they should remain cognizant that such behavior—like erotic asphyxiation—can result in permanent brain injury or death.

Besides the possibility of death to the entire body, both "fainting game" and erotic asphyxiation can kill extensive amounts of brain cells, thereby causing permanent impairments in neurological functions. According to some studies published by the National Vital Statistics System, more than 85 percent of those who died from such behaviors were males—mostly in their early teens.

Because such instances are reportedly widespread throughout our society, physicians need to follow the recommendations of the Centers for Disease Control. These guidelines urge doctors to be on the lookout for early warning signs of such behaviors, such as bloodshot eyes, disorientation, spending lots of time alone, and severe headaches.

Some People Yearn For Painful Spankings

Strangely, at least from the perspective of us people who lack such predilections, some individuals crave and desperately yearn to receive painful spankings. And, oddly enough, just as many people desire to inflict such punishments as well.

"Every normal person, in fact, is only normal on the average," said Sigmund Freud, the famed neurologist and founder of a school of psychiatry in the late 19th Century and early 20th Century. "His ego approximates to that of the psychotic in some part or other, and to a greater or lesser extent."

Freud has been just one of a vast array of psychiatric and behavioral experts who have presented numerous diverse theories on what motivates some individuals to eagerly receive or to inflict pain. Suggestions have spanned the gambit from troubled childhoods, hidden yearnings to gain attention from a parent-like figure, or even secret sexual preferences.

The general term of S&M for sadism and masochism is also linked to the phenomenon of bondage and discipline, sometimes called B&D or "dominance and submission." When combined as an overall lifestyle practice, these various terms are sometimes referred to by the moniker "BDSM."

Locked in today's era of political correctness, some practitioners of the BDSM lifestyle complain that any attempt to label and scientifically explain their behaviors is unfair or even hurtful—if you will pardon the pun.

Whatever the reasons for such motivations, many of us from the general population find ourselves puzzled and even mortified by such behaviors. And, from the standpoint of law enforcement, any defense argument that the victim "wanted this," or "it was consensual" would fall on deaf ears—since the law refuses to view such proclamations as justifiable or warranted when death or severe injury becomes the result.

Any Yearning for Pain Confuses Some People

Individuals now suffering from extreme pain caused by diseases or afflictions such as cancer, arthritis or tooth decay might find themselves repulsed by the very notion that other people actually crave extreme pain or even bondage-style confinement.

Yes, our brains and ultimately our personal motivations and desires serve as key, integral tools in determining whether we want to ward off or eagerly receive physical pain. Thus, the magnetism for— or the repulsion against—such sensations is at the center of the proverbial bull's-eye that medical professionals seek to identify and target worldwide.

"A day spent without the sight or sound of beauty, the contemplation of mystery, or the search of truth or perfection is a poverty-stricken day; and a succession of such days is fatal to human life," said Lewis Mumford, a 20th Century American historian and philosopher.

According to various published accounts, a fairly high percentage of people in the modern U.S. culture have yearned for and participated at least once in the process of bondage, enduring the psychological pain of being physically constrained. This desire is sometimes attributed to a yearning to have someone in a position of trust take a dominant role.

Those of us within the medical profession should always remain fully cognizant that many of our patients—but not all of them— look to us for seasoned leadership and knowledge. While a patient's psychological preference on a personal level should never get confused with the proper diagnostic process and eventually treatment, in almost every case mental factors and motivations play a huge role.

"Both the man of science and the man of action live always at the edge of mystery, surrounded by it," said Julius "J" Robert Oppenheimer, a 20th Century American theoretical physicist.

Chapter 18

Some Use Humor as a Coping Mechanism

The mere notion of physical pain digs so deeply into the human psyche that people often use humor in an effort to cope with such sensations or even to alleviate the resulting mental anguish.

At times such entertainment has even blossomed to the point where movie and TV audiences roar in laughter, upon seeing popular characters killed or seriously injured.

Commonly called dark comedy, dark humor or black comedy, such films, stage shows or books strive to put everything from murder to barbarism and even disabilities into a funny light. Through the early 1900s film stars that featured painful situations to generate laughs included everyone from Charlie Chaplain to Buster Keaton, Harold Lloyd, the Marx Brothers and the Three Stooges.

Long before he became a film star, Keaton began performing in comical stage shows at age 3 along with his father, Joseph Hallie "Joe" Keaton. As the 20th Century began, audiences of this traveling show roared in laughter whenever the father threw his disobedient son against scenery, into the orchestra pit and even into the audience.

Since these scenes were well-rehearsed and highly choreographed, the child always escaped injury. Yet unsuspecting audiences adored

the boy's comical expressions, which sparked the indomitable human spirit within show-goers who witnessed first-hand that a person can endure and even persevere through physically painful situations.

"I've simply been brought up being knocked down," said Keaton, who died in 1966 at age 70. Throughout his life, with varying degrees of intermittent success, Keaton was among those who benefited financially from the yearnings of others to witness the calamities that befall those of us who suffer physical pain.

People Invariably Want to Beat Pain

Throughout my many years as a physician, I have personally witnessed countless instances where people bravely faced horrific pain—often resorting to humor as a powerful weapon to help alleviate their mental and physical anguish.

By their very nature, the vast majority of people are "fighters" who yearn to win and to persevere through the midst of real or perceived hardships. Yes, Mother Nature commands that we struggle to remain alive and stay vibrant for as long as possible. And, for the most part, humor invariably plays an integral role in helping to enable at least some of us to cope with these struggles.

In the blockbuster 1999 comic film "Patch Adams," superstar Robin Williams played a widely acclaimed real-life American physician, Hunter Doherty "Patch" Adams. Also an active author and social activist, Adams organized volunteers who traveled the world—dressed as clowns for entertaining patients, orphans and many other people.

Although Adams has been quoted as criticizing the film for portraying him as merely a funny doctor, there is no denying that humor and basic entertainment such as the shows he organized can go a long way toward helping people alleviate, ignore, or cope with pain—while also encouraging patients to take the path to eventual recovery.

Fully cognizant of the need to keep humor as an essential ingredient toward recovery, my professional medical and office staff maintains video tapes and discs of movies including many popular comedies. While many of my patients receive intravenous treatments such as certain chemotherapies or immune boosters, they often eagerly seize the opportunity to watch the films.

Film Star Harold Lloyd Helped Lead the Way

Silent film star Harold Lloyd made significant strides in enabling people to laugh at extremely painful situations, even suffering a horrendous real-life hand injury during the 1919 filming of "Haunted Spooks"—losing a thumb and index finger in a bomb blast. The injury forced Lloyd to wear a prosthetic glove in subsequent films, including "Safety Last" in 1923 where his character dangles from the bending hands of a clock near the top of a skyscraper. Nervous but excited audiences roared in laughter.

The legendary silent film star Charlie Chaplain also delighted fans in classic films such as "The Gold Rush" in 1925, where his beloved "Tramp" character dangles from a cabin at the precipice of a cliff in the Klondike, battles an escaped fugitive, and carves a nail-lined boot in hopes of enjoying a tasty meal.

The reasons why people laugh hysterically at potentially painful situations may stem at least in part from the intensity of emotions we all instinctively know that such sensations often elicit. And, of course, the potential for great humor often seems to intensify when the danger threatens other people rather than us—particularly to our perceived enemies or to individuals that we care little or nothing about.

Although failing to perform well at the box office, the Marx Brothers' 1933 anarchic film "Duck Soup" is now considered among history's greatest comedy movies as listed by the American Film Institute. Groucho Marx portrays Rufus T. Firefly, a character some observers say seemed loosely modeled after the Italian fascist Benito Mussolini—who actually ended up banning the film in that nation. The plot ridicules the absurdity of war and its resulting pain, death, injuries and destruction.

After starting their own successful act on Vaudeville, The Three Stooges spread their slapstick comedy worldwide in films distributed worldwide. Their comedy brand fit the mold of slapstick, where exaggerated violence greatly exceeded what most people would consider common sense. Their characters would go overboard, such as hitting each other over the head with hammers or throwing their adversaries or each other to the floor.

John Deszo Ratzenberger, an American actor and star of the hit 1980s CBS-TV sitcom "Cheers," has been quoted as saying that "a farce, or slapstick humor, does well universally." Indeed, almost every culture invariably knows and appreciates the universal sensation of physical pain and even mental anguish.

James W. Forsythe, M.D., H.M.D.

Use Slapstick Humor to Battle our Own Actual Pains

Historians tell us that the use of slapstick humor prevailed in many cultures through Europe and eventually the Americas beginning as far back as the Renaissance and even the Middle Ages. Some history buffs even argue that slapstick or dark humor sometimes even emerged as a key factor in Greek and Roman stage productions thousands of years ago. Today, while remaining fully cognizant that slapstick humor is pure farce, people suffering from severe pain can face their afflictions head-on—perhaps even erupting in a healthy laugh at their own current predicaments.

Even the great, unsurpassable bard Shakespeare in the late 1500s and early 1600s penned gripping, uproarious comedies that featured chase scenes with painful consequences and beatings. Perhaps the most notable among them in terms of slapstick, puns and mistaken identity was among his first works, "The Comedy of Errors." The plot even delves into such normally delicate topics as demonic possession, theft and even infidelity.

Some noted thespians even go so far as to say that in creating this production, Shakespeare used as his primary models two plays written in the second century before Christ by Titus Maccius Plautus. These ancient works marked the early beginnings of the slapstick genre, which gained widespread popularity in the American culture in the 1900s thanks largely to entertainment by such greats as Laurel and Hardy, and the Keystone Kops.

At the height of their own real-life discomforts, many people might consider the very idea of laughing at pain as unthinkable or perhaps

159

even offensive. The paradoxical nature of such dueling mental motivations and opposite perspectives could very well confuse even the most seasoned practitioners of psychiatric medicine. Nonetheless, perhaps because human nature makes many of us want to laugh at pain, slapstick-style entertainment also blossomed into the arena of animated films.

In popular "Tom and Jerry" cartoon shorts and features, comic violence often prevailed in non-stop chases and battles—usually when Tom the cat unsuccessfully tried to trap Jerry the mouse. Sometimes audiences laughed with the greatest intensity when the productions were pushed to the limits of socially acceptable gore, such as when Jerry works to cut Tom in half. The cat employed a wide array of tools, weapons and everyday household objects, from waffle irons and refrigerators to mallets.

The "Wile E. Coyote and the Roadrunner" animations also features slapstick comedy, especially when the coyote develops elaborate but eventually unsuccessful plans to capture or eliminate the bird. This animation's character creator, Chuck Jones, has been quoted as saying he based the coyote on a similar creature from Mark Twain's "Roughing It."

Chapter 19

Video Game Entertainment Sometimes Goes Too Far

The basic entertainment of stage, music, radio, movies and TV has expanded in recent decades to include video games. Many of these creations are hinged on violence, in which participants strive to inflict horribly painful wounds on various animated characters.

Although many video games are peaceful or intellectually based puzzles, from the view of many critics far too many of these devices delve more than necessary into the realm of pain and needless or senseless violence. Opponents complain that besides being addictive to some individuals, especially boys in their early or middle teens, such games might tend to make participants insensitive to the pains suffered by other human beings.

Shigeru Miyamoto, a Japanese designer of video games, has been quoted as saying that "video games are bad for you? That's what they said about rock 'n' roll."

Some politicians and educators take offense to such observations, especially those who worry that some people who enjoy violent video games might tend to become overly aggressive in real-life situations.

From my view, while entertainment in general—and even some forms of slapstick—serve as healthy distractions from physical pain and mental anguish, the excessive use of violent video games could cause far more harm than good for participants. Of course, many proponents of these games argue that absolutely no correlation can be found in such on-screen activities and highly aggressive real-world violence.

All along, some observers also note the scientists lack reliable, comprehensive studies on the issue. A 2001 article in "Psychological Science" questions whether youths who play such games tend to become violent. Even so, reports in numerous other respected medical publications such as the "Journal of Adolescent Health" from Harvard Medical School's Center for Mental Health find no correlation between actual violence and such games.

Some politicians have even pushed for legislation that would ban such entertainment, moves that have sparked the ire of those who argue that such laws would violate the free speech of participants.

Ultimately, at least from my view, this primal issue boils down to the fact that inborn, natural instinct motivates many people— particularly teenagers within their vital formative years—to experiment or participate in actions that could result in pain. The key here is for parents to actively monitor the activities of their children, and to impose restrictions or professional intervention when such activities become extreme.

Punk Rock Also Glorifies the Suffering of Pain

Some observers might even argue that the punk rock music and entertainment genre glorifies and thrives in a glorification of physical pain and mental anguish.

Although some observers might argue otherwise, this genre embraced a rebellious over-the-edge lifestyles when first bursting onto the scene in the 1970s. This music's wild, rebellious focus and the resulting atmosphere might have contributed to the early suicide deaths of such stars as Sid Vicious of the Sex Pistols punk rock band.

In the eyes of many observers and fans, such music and the genre's most popular performers conveyed a clear, distinct message that life is meaningless, pointless and without any significant purpose. And, a big part of this atmosphere conveyed a sense that the world is filled with relentless pain.

Many young people worldwide embraced this "nothing matters" lifestyle, even after Sid Vicious, a native of England, died in New York City of an apparent heroin overdose at age 21 in February 1979.

Nearly two decades later the grunge music scene brought fame to such stars as Kurt Cobain, found dead at age 27 in April 1994 of suicide by gunshot. An autopsy indicated heroin and valium in his body. Some musicologists describe grunge as hardcore punk or a heavy metal style of independent rock, like standard punk filled with lyrics and tones denoting angst and apathy to the endless pain the world imposes on us all.

As if seeming apathetic and even disassociated with the chronic mental pain and anguish he suffered in his personal life, Cobain was once quoted as saying that "If you die, you're completely happy, and your soul somewhere lives on. I'm not afraid of dying. Total peace after death, becoming someone else is the best hope I've got."

Today, people worldwide suffering from such maladies as advanced-stage cancer or AIDS might find themselves repulsed by such attitudes, the notion that some people consider life itself—let alone the pain we all must endure—as meaningless.

Other celebrities and everyday common people have shunned the notion of tragedy or pain for much different reasons. Even "The King of Rock" Elvis Presley, who died at age 42 in 1977 of apparent heart complications exacerbated in part by the abuse of painkillers, was once quoted as saying that "I have no use for bodyguards, but I have very specific use for highly trained certified public accountants."

Alice Cooper Prospered in the Musical Pain Business

Enthralled, evil-minded, bloodthirsty audiences swamped to worldwide performances of Alice Cooper, a rock 'n' roll star whose popularity skyrocketed in the early 1970s, after his live stage music shows began featuring many painful scenes.

Many of Cooper's most ardent fans appreciated the shock value of his numerous pain-oriented stage theatrics, everything from an electric chair, guillotines and gallows to boa constrictors, blood and baby dolls.

Some of Cooper's greatest notoriety stemmed from mainstream news media reports that he had apparently bitten the head off a live chicken and drunk its blood during a live stage show. According to some published reports, other rock stars had privately urged Cooper never to deny the incident even if it were untrue.

Yes, more than 2,000 years after gladiators clashed at the Coliseum in Rome and 500 years after the sacrifice of tens of thousands of people the future Mexico City's early Aztec culture, many people still yearned to witness live, gory, painful scenes.

"I object to violence, because when it appears to do good, the good is only temporary. The evil it does is permanent," said Mohandas Gandhi, a spiritual leader who embraced non-violent activism in India's independence movement of the 20th Century.

Despite such peace-oriented philosophies, rock stars like Cooper thrived upon and embraced almost any shocking theatrics that communicated a sense of overwhelming pain. Indeed, as Cooper once admitted to the media, "We were once into fun, sex, death, and money, while everyone else was into peace and love."

To those of us who become personally gratified and fulfilled by caring for other people, such seemingly heartless motivations boggle the mind. Still, upon careful observation, we must admit to ourselves that at least for the foreseeable future many entertainers such as Cooper will seek to prosper from some of the worst aspects of the human psyche. For anyone who truly believes that ultimately "good always triumphs over evil," a relentless hope remains that good, loving and motivational entertainment forms will prevail.

Positive Entertainment Can Play a Significant Role

One of my many great personal heroes has been the late legendary American comic Bob Hope, who died in 2003 at age 100. From

World War II, and the Korean War through the Vietnam War and well beyond, Hope brought much-needed humor and lively stage shows to our nation's troops. These energetic productions brought vital distractions and even some much-needed laughs to soldiers and sailors amid the heat of battle. Hope and his show biz entourage entertained me and my fellow soldiers in Vietnam in 1969.

Since the Second World War, the United Service Organizations, commonly known as the USO, has helped take an essential lead role in addressing the vital need to bring entertainment to our troops who face relentless mental and physical pain. From my personal perspective, along with those of many other physicians, the USO has played a vital role in helping to give both healthy troops and those suffering from painful injuries the positive-minded spirit and motivations necessary to endure and persevere.

Besides Hope, the many entertainers who volunteered their precious time and entertainment services included Wayne Newton and Jayne Mansfield, to Redd Foxx, Marilyn Monroe, Nancy Sinatra, John Wayne, Ann-Margaret, and many others.

In fact, historians tell us that varying forms of entertainment have played a vital role in many wars, serving as an attempt to distract soldiers and even their loved ones from physical and emotional pains. Less than a few weeks after the official end of the Civil War, President Abraham Lincoln was fatally shot on April 14, 1865, by actor John Wilkes at Ford's Theater in Washington, D.C., where many people had presumably sought entertainment as a distraction from the prevalent worries and pains of the time.

"America is addicted to the wars of distraction," said Barbara Ehrenreich, an American political activist and essayist.

Sociologists tell us that the very nature of entertainment serves as a form of distraction from our everyday lives. This process can sometimes take our minds away from other worries and stresses, key among them anything to do with mental or physical pain.

Chapter 20

Pets Also Can Play an Integral Role in Fighting Pain

Seasoned physicians and medical professionals from many specialties have learned the increasing importance that pets can play in helping us to alleviate pain or physical discomforts. Widely respected and much-needed organizations such as Therapy Dogs United have brought a positive impact to the lives of patients in hospitals and individuals as they undergo essential physical therapies.

With increased frequency in recent years, hospitals and other important medical facilities nationwide have accepted the vital services of such volunteers. Trained or obedient dogs and cats sometimes serve essential roles in what medial professionals call animal-assisted therapy.

The primary objectives of such pet owners who volunteer their time and energy are to assist patients in improving their cognitive skills, social interactions, physical abilities and emotional well being. Significant improvement in any or all these areas can go a long way in helping to eliminate both physical and emotional pain.

Many such programs require that before being accepted the pets must undergo rigorous veterinary examinations to help ensure the animals are healthy enough for such activities, while also avoiding the likelihood of spreading diseases.

Besides dogs and cats, according to a variety of published accounts the various species recruited to assist in such efforts range from elephants and llamas to lizards and rabbits.

Volunteers Make Extraordinary Contributions

Every day, nationwide and around the world volunteers bring their animals to hospitals, medical clinics and physical therapy facilities for interaction with human patients.

Besides helping patients improve their abilities to move about freely, a process that medical experts call "motor skills," via animal-assisted therapy some patients also can enjoy improvements in their abilities to stand or to use mobility devices like wheelchairs.

Just as impressive, according to some research this process also sometimes goes a long way toward enabling patients to improve their self-esteem, while helping to reduce anxiety and loneliness. All along, some patients even re-learn the ability to trust.

Although some observers have called such therapies nothing more than a "dangerous fad," many medical professionals ardently believe such efforts provide essential value in the process of striving for physical and mental improvements.

Whether this process inspires or motivates participation in group activities, and improves interactions with others apparently remain questions for continued study. All along, many of those who participate in such activities insist the process has definite value.

According to one age-old saying about pets, "One reason a dog can be such a comfort when you're feeling blue is that he doesn't try to find out why." Those who embrace and encourage animal-assisted therapies encourage such observations.

"Animals are such agreeable friends," said Mary Anne Evans, the 19th Century English novelist who wrote under the pen name George Eliot. "They ask no questions; they pass no criticisms."

Animal-Assisted Therapy Has a Vibrant History

Many advocates of animal-assisted therapies insist the process has an important and vibrant history. According to some published accounts, a U.S. Army soldier, Corporal William Wynne, was often visited by a Yorkshire terrier, "Smoky," while the man recovered at a hospital in the Philippines during World War II.

Dr. Charles Mayo, namesake of the internationally acclaimed Mayo Clinic in Rochester, Minn., began taking Smoky on his rounds after the dog became increasingly popular among patients in the Philippines hospital. The dog emerged as a hit among patients and staffers, motivating them to continue using the pet in the therapy process for a 12-year period through the war and afterward.

Advocates using animals such as Smoky insisted that these visits helped reduce stress experienced by individual patients. As Doctor

Mayo observed, "worry affects the circulation, the heart, the glands, the whole nervous system, and profoundly affects heart action."

Medical professionals in other parts of the globe also independently recognized the many benefits generated by visits from animals. In England, registered nurse Elaine Smith noticed improvements in patients after visits from a chaplain accompanied by his golden retriever. Inspired by these improvements, Smith returned to the United States, where she launched programs for training dogs for such visits.

While seeing-eye dogs have been used to assist the blind for many generations, it wasn't until recent decades that some medical facilities began actively recruiting dogs for use when striving to enable children to overcome emotional or speech disorders.

Chapter 21

Human Beings Cause Pain as Relentless Parasites

By some accounts, human being are the most prodigious, efficient and biologically successfully parasites in world history. In nature, most parasites are much smaller than the hosts that they live off of, sometimes eating at the very creatures that they specialize in and depend on for survival.

Some people might argue that human beings are biological "parasites" as well, at least in the sense that we virtually live off of many thousands of other animals to survive.

Think of it this way. Since the moment you were born, virtually everything you have eaten in order to grow, to thrive and to remain alive was at one time a living creature—either a plant or an animal.

For the vast majority of people, this means that many hundreds or more likely literally thousands of animals have died painful or uncomfortable deaths, just so that each of us can remain alive.

And, whether we like to face this fact or not, a vast majority of the animals that we eat in the form of fish, poultry or meat products suffered at least some physical pain during the slaughtering process.

Even the turkeys that we are so thankful for at our Thanksgiving or holiday meals suffered at least some discomfort, often during a decapitation process.

Meantime, a debate persists among scientists on whether plants can feel or at least sense physical pain. Some observers call such a notion pure bunk, since plants lack the brains and central nervous systems that convey such sensations. Yet other critics claim plants sense or experience pain, plus basic reactions to environmental conditions.

In any case, there is no denying that so you could remain alive today, creatures from many species have died from among both plant and animal species. Lots of these creatures depend on us for their survival and for being created in the first place. In many cases, these various individuals ranging from plants to animals would never have existed without us and— depending on specific environmental and social conditions—we depend on them for survival as well.

Slaughterhouses Thrive So that We Can Live

At this very moment, whether we like the fact or not, many thousands of animals are in the process of being destroyed in the food-production process. According to scientists and slaughterhouse professionals, in most cases only 45 percent to 50 percent of each cattle carcass is edible. Any remaining materials are often used for various other byproducts such as leather and soap.

The process is so huge that by some estimates just more than a half million people work in the animal destruction and processing business. This killing system enables many of us to remain gainfully employed. But, there is no escaping that for the most part, the process usually involves pain or at least some discomfort for the animals involved.

More than 28 billion pounds of beef are processed every year in the United States alone, according to the U.S. Department of Agriculture. And, more than 650 million animals are killed yearly in Canada.

Due largely to the massive amounts of necessary killing, some analysts insist the process is cost-effective and efficient only when the animals are slaughtered and butchered as fast as possible. From the view of animal rights advocates this sometimes causes oversights or downright greedy tactics that inflict unnecessary pain and suffering on the condemned.

Citing ethical concerns, some vegetarians join animal rights advocates in sharply criticizing the slaughter. Despite these concerns, the intentional, methodical, relentless and never-ending killing of animals is likely to continue for a long time to come. After all, large segments of the earth's population crave, need and demand such foods no matter how much pain the slaughtering system might entail.

All along, operators of some animal processing facilities report that they're making focused, concerted efforts to address such concerns. Newly designed and constructed entrances at some facilities prevent livestock from seeing or realizing the fate that awaits them. Many slaughterhouses render cattle unconscious via electric shock, prior to the severing of vital arteries or veins by knife.

Laws and customs regulating or mandating the methods of animal slaughter vary worldwide. In the U.S., the Humane Slaughter Act of 1958 requires that horses, swine, sheep and cattle get just one application of a stunning device. Some advocates insist that when done properly by highly trained slaughterhouse technicians the stunning involves little or no pain in a relatively stress-free environment.

However, some publications have quoted slaughterhouse workers as saying that the massive quantities of animals and the necessary speed of processing sometimes results in instances where animals are skinned alive—kicking and shrieking at the moment of death.

Chapter 22

Selfishness, Ignorance and Apathy Result in Pollution-Caused Pain

R eckless and ignoring the health of others, people and industries worldwide cause widespread pollution that ultimately instigates extremely painful diseases.

Some sociologists and economic experts might blame this problem primarily on overcrowding, as the Earth's population approaches and surpasses 7 billion people. According to recent news reports, the crush of human beings also has played a key role in igniting super-high grocery prices and even "food riots" in numerous continents.

"Our lives are to be used and thus to be lived as fully as possible, and truly it seems that we are never so alive as when we concern ourselves with other people," said Harry Chapin, an American singer in the 1900s.

Despite such good-intentioned philosophies, entire societies and huge corporations worldwide have inflicted intense physical pain on many individuals by creating and carelessly spreading carcinogenic pollutions.

Excessive levels of foreign, harmful substances have been pumped into the atmosphere, driven into the soils of vital croplands, and pumped needlessly throughout essential water supplies—including the very oceans on which much of the world's ecosystem depends.

Historians tell us that the propensity of human beings to generate harmful pollutants began hundreds or perhaps even thousands of years ago. Startled anthropologists have found harmful levels of soot on the ceilings of prehistoric caves, and scientists also have discovered evidence of potentially harmful levels of metals produced long ago by the ancient Chinese, Greeks and Romans.

"There is nothing more frightful than ignorance in action," said Johann Wolfgang von Goethe, a German novelist, playwright and poet in the 18th and 19th Centuries.

Societies and diverse cultures worldwide have openly acknowledged the harmfulness of pollution for more than 1,000 years, sometimes taking governmental measures in fruitless efforts to ban or regulate the processing and disposal of pain-causing substances. In 1272, concerned by increasingly harmful smoke, King Edward I of England prohibited the inhabitants of his kingdom from burning sea coal. Yet air pollution persisted in Great Britain, particularly during the Great Smog of 1952.

These are just a handful of the countless examples of widespread environmental damage on the international scale, sparking extremely painful afflictions such as lung disease and slow-killing cancers that ravage the body's vital organs. These problems worsened with the advent of the industrial revolution in the late 1800s and early 1900s, when massive building, energy-producing and mining projects kicked into full gear at a previously unheard of magnitude.

James W. Forsythe, M.D., H.M.D.

The Ignorance of Humans Transitioned into the Nuclear Age

The emergence of nuclear technology in the mid-1900s sparked selfish, mindless and ill-advised testing that instilled fatal and extremely painful cancers in thousands of people.

The vast majority of those suffering from fatal cancers as a result of nuclear bomb tests in the Nevada desert were relatively unknown, everyday folks whose names almost never reached the mainstream news media.

But at least one incident involved dozens of celebrities, movie stars unlucky enough to be on a Utah movie set in a wilderness area upwind from nuclear radiation spread by an atomic bomb blast in the neighboring Silver State.

All major stars from the 1956 CinemaScope® epic movie "The Conqueror" about Genghis Khan, featuring John Wayne, Rita Hayworth, Agnes Moorehead and Pedro Armendáriz, eventually suffered from fatal cancer. The movie's director, Dick Powell, also an actor, suffered a similar fate.

According to some published reports, a whopping 91 of the total 220 people from the film's cast and crew contracted extremely painful and often-fatal cancers by the early 1980s. Numerous reports through the years have claimed that under normal circumstances only 30 people from the total 220 individuals would have suffered from cancer during their lifetimes.

Powell died in 1963, the same year that Armendáriz committed suicide after learning he had incurable kidney cancer. Wayne,

Hayworth and Moorehead all died in the 1970s. Skeptics have noted that Wayne and Moorehead were heavy smokers, and that cancers instilled by exposure to radiation lack lengthy incubation periods, the time that elapses between a person's exposure to a chemical, radiation or organism.

Through the late 1990s, thousands of people in the western United States contracted cancer that some critics attribute to fallout from the nuclear bomb tests. And, at least 4,000 deaths have been attributed the April 1986 Chernobyl disaster, when a nuclear power plant malfunctioned in the Ukraine; many Chernobyl victims suffered long, drawn-out and excruciatingly painful deaths caused by cancers attributed to nuclear radiation. Various news reports stated that more than 25,000 were killed in 2011 in Japan's major earthquake, tsunami and radiation disaster.

"It's no use reminding yourself daily that you are mortal; it will be brought home to you soon enough," said Albert Camus, the 20th Century French novelist, essayist and playwright.

Pollutants Often Generate Carcinogens

As an integrative medical oncologist, every day I treat patients from around the world who suffer from excruciatingly painful cancers— many of which were likely caused by carcinogens generated by harmful pollutants. Needless to say, much of the time the physical pains sometimes generate mental anguish or stresses as well.

Technically, scientists classify a "carcinogen" as any substance that directly causes cancer by damaging certain cellular structures within a person's body. Researchers have identified many types of carcinogens, some that naturally occur in the environment and others that result from human activities such as the generation of certain radiations.

By the time many of my patients first arrive at my clinic, some after traveling more than 10,000 miles, they already know the basic types of cancers they suffer from following an initial diagnosis performed elsewhere. Amid their initial visits with my professional staff, most patients are well past the point of worrying about what caused their ailment. At this point, they're focused on receiving treatments or what some refer to as a possible "cure."

In addition, a small percentage of my patients do not suffer from cancer but instead from a variety of other physical ailments that some attribute to pollutants or contaminants that damage the body's immune systems. Some of these conditions result in extremely painful symptoms.

Walter Matthau, an American comic movie star who reached the height of his popularity in the 20th Century, once joked that "my doctor gave me six months to live, but when I couldn't pay the bill he gave me six months more."

Without exaggeration, along with the assistance and persistence of my highly trained, knowledgeable and professional staff, I continually strive to give each of my patients hope for effective treatments and the possible eradication of their pains and illnesses.

And, for those who happen to ask, I sometimes cite or list the possible causes of their cancers or other ailments. As you might imagine, lots of patients find themselves startled to discover that at least in some instances their painful medical conditions might be no fault of their own—but rather a result of adverse environmental substances such as toxic metals, pollutants, harmful chemicals or various forms of radiation.

The long list of naturally occurring carcinogens, some which are pushed together in limited spaces or pumped out in massive quantities in the industrial process, include asbestos, a naturally occurring silicate mineral; benzene, an organic chemical compound; toxic dioxins, numerous substances each with varying degrees of toxicity; and many others including kepone, once commonly used as an insecticide.

The many other carcinogens that people often ignorantly or mindlessly inflict on themselves or others include tobacco smoke; formaldehyde, sometimes used in the embalming or plastics-making processes; and vinyl chloride, often used in the production of specific plastics used in everything from clothes to garden hoses.

Food Preparation Methods Can Generate Carcinogens

Do you know that by preparing or cooking certain foods the "wrong" way, you can inadvertently create carcinogens that generate extremely painful or even deadly cancers? Well, this actually happens according to some studies and in such cases the cook or restaurant mindlessly, carelessly or ignorantly generates disease.

Scientists tell us many potent carcinogens get generated in minute quantities in specific instances where foods are cooked at excessively high temperatures, such as in the grilling or barbecuing process.

If this actually occurs as some medical professionals claim, then we have yet another lifestyle behavior where people either recklessly or inadvertently inflict potentially painful conditions on others.

Meantime, various other medical reports indicate that overheating or frying in the processes of cooking various carbohydrate foods such as French fries and potato chips sometimes generates a known animal carcinogen.

As researchers continue studying and pinpointing these various potential or possible risks, all of us need to keep in mind that sometimes people create painful conditions while fully unaware of such implications—rather than any "ignorant" failure to perform adequate research or testing beforehand.

Some People Knowingly Spread Infectious Diseases

Worsening the danger, throughout history some people have either knowingly or willfully spread or exposed other individuals to extremely painful or even fatal infectious diseases. According to various charity reports, at least 33 million people worldwide in 2009 were infected with HIV, the usually fatal viral infection causing AIDS or Acquired Immune Deficiency Syndrome. Each year, according to these estimates, more than 2 million people contract AIDS, which often results in extremely painful medical conditions ranging from cancer to weakened immunity and resistant severe infections—bacterial, viral, fungal and parasitic.

Yet officials apparently have no conclusive estimate on how many of these people contracted the disease after other individuals either knowingly or recklessly exposed these victims to the virus—often spread via sexual contact.

However, we can say with certainty that almost daily news reports from various communities worldwide describe arrests and convictions of HIV-infected people who knowingly or willfully engaged in sex with other individuals—without telling the victims that they had the disease.

Such horrific news signals to us all that merely for their own sexual gratification, some people are willing to expose others to the possibility of extremely painful disease or even death. Numerous cases involve HIV-infected individuals who knowingly or eagerly engage in unprotected sex with dozens or even hundreds of people.

Such insensitivity brings to mind the old saying that "all good things must come to an end, but all bad things can continue forever." The undeniable, relentless and persistent fact that all life involves at least some degree of pain either gets microscopic treatment or totally ignored in such conditions.

The American freelance journalist and satirist Chuck Palahniuk has been quoted as saying that "it's easy to cry when you realize that everyone you love will reject you or die." From my personal view, the propensity for emotional grief intensifies when we take into account that the many similarities between love and pain often get intermixed, creating ugliness for some people within a world that should be filled with great joy.

Determined to blast a crack through the proverbial face of such cruelty and selfishness, I urge all patients—no matter how hopeless a medical situation might seem—to take a positive view in the direction of envisioned or planned good results. Yes, as some of the world's wisest leaders have said, "Smile, even if it's a sad smile, sadder than a sad smile is the sadness of not knowing how to smile."

Painful Infectious Diseases Have Persevered

Despite numerous significant and noteworthy advances in modern medicine, many specific types of painful and sometimes fatal infectious diseases persist across the United States and worldwide.

Each day, people get the mortifying news that they or their loved ones are suffering from these afflictions. The many diseases or viruses range from the flu and gastrointestinal maladies to cholera and Rocky Mountain Spotted Fever.

Measles, the chicken pox and the mumps also make the list of dreaded maladies. Thanks to medical advances, some of the most feared diseases have been eradicated, including smallpox—which, by some estimates caused from 300 million to 500 million deaths during the 20th Century.

Meantime, the development of a polio vaccine during the 1950s eliminated much of the dreaded, crippling polio; physicians and charitable organizations hope to eventually eradicate the disease worldwide using these medicines. Bill Gates, the billionaire founder of Microsoft, announced in 2011 that he has given hundreds of millions of dollars to a charity designed to permanently wipe out polio worldwide.

Chapter 23

Developing Pain Relievers Took Creativity

Since the beginning of recorded history, varying societies have created diverse belief systems, remedies and technologies in a variety of medical systems—mostly with the primary goal of relieving pain. Many cultures attributed physical pains, severe illness and mental stresses on the presumed or supposed "will of the gods."

Just as interesting, numerous societies hundreds or thousands of years ago also cited everything from witchcraft to the positioning of stars for the emergence of certain painful conditions. Such prevalent beliefs in such systems gradually faded for the most part thanks to the eventual advent and emergence of modern science.

Various published reports conclude that historians have been unable to pinpoint any verifiable, irrefutable written records that designate specifically which herbs early humans first used in efforts to alleviate or eliminate pain.

Anthropologists classify "prehistoric medicine" as any pain-relieving and illness remedies that the world's many cultures used before people invented writing. According to a "Health Guidance" article published in 2009, a considerable variety of early cultures cited or believed in natural and supernatural reasons for illness. And, numerous cultures used similar overall methods in attempts at cures or perceived remedies.

Often blaming sorcery, the gods or even spirits perceived as evil, these diverse cultures from Native Americans to native people on other continents developed widely diverse methods of treating or dealing with individuals suffering from diseases.

The Cherokee and Navaho tribes in early North America used kindness in treating people who were disabled or deformed, the "Health Guidance" article says. However, the same story also points out that Eskimos in the extreme north put elderly people in unsheltered icy areas when food supplies dwindled. And some Native American cultures accepted the suicides of their mature tribe members, often a "means of removing the burden of their dependence."

Perhaps these once-prevalent practices disappeared or at least dissipated as many people within these cultures gradually realized— individually and collectively—that such cruelties proved fruitless, resulting in little or no benefit to their cultures.

"A science that does not bring us nearer to God is worthless," said Simone Weil, a French social philosopher and mystic in the early 20th Century.

Early Purveyors of Healing Were Often Called "Medicine Men"

Anthropologists and sociologists tell us that many pre-historic cultures from such diverse regions as North America to the Congo almost always invariably looked to a single, central figure for advice or to take action in the hoped-for healing process. To the North American tribes, these individuals were often hailed as the "medicine man." To Eskimos and Siberians, such individuals were "shamans," while some jungle-based cultures such as those in the Congo referred to these individuals as "witch doctors."

Many tribes or clans looked to one individual to handle the essential role of eliminating pain or curing illness; other societies or cultures sought the help of a group of healers formed within secret societies. Certain individuals were allowed into these positions or groups only after demonstrating that they had experienced persistent dreams about possible remedies or reasons for illness. Other recruits sometimes displayed psychic powers perceived as strong. Also, numerous individuals entrusted in such positions had displayed a strong desire to fill these posts.

"In virtually none of these primitive societies was entrance into this vocation taken lightly," Health Guidance said. "Among American Indians and also in the African Congo, a doctor could amass wealth but also was vulnerable to attack if his medicine was 'bad'—that is, if he did not utilize the accepted methods. The outcome did not always have to be successful, but the techniques were expected to be above reproach."

Perhaps these overall ancient, antiquated requirements mirror at least in part much of today's mainstream allopathic medical practices, including methods that sometimes are considered mandatory although the techniques are ineffective. A key example might be the excessive or unnecessary employment of extreme levels of chemotherapies, even in instances where standard science and historic results indicate such treatments provide little or no effective results.

"Resignation—not mystic, not detached—but resignation open-eyed, conscious and informed by love is the only one of our feelings for which it is impossible to become a sham," said Joseph Conrad, an English novelist in the late 19th Century and early 20th Century.

Today's Medicine Has Vast but Specifically Defined Objectives

Unlike the physicians of today, the mystics, medicine men, witch doctors and shamans of the past also were occasionally or prevalently held responsible for everything from the daily weather to the vibrancy of crops within their cultures.

While today's many medical specialties range from oncology to urology and many more categories, some early cultures had specialists in everything from dealing with unexpected catastrophes to performing specific types of religious rites. Anthropologists insist the advent of herbs designed to treat pain gradually emerged into many of these various societies, in some cases thousands of years ago.

The job of casting magical spells fell on sorcerers, and many cultures looked to soothsayers for predicting future events. At least in a sense these responsibilities carry over into the modern era, where some doctors are expected to perform as if miracle workers and some patients demand accurate, long-term prognosis on the progression of—or the likely outcome of—an individual's diseases.

Such great and sometimes unrealistic expectations often leave many of today's most talented physicians and medical professionals in a cautious mode, particularly in instances that involve well-intentioned

attempts to relieve or eliminate extreme pain.
"I am not in this world to live up to other people's expectations, nor do I feel that the world must live up to mine," said Fritz Perls, a 20th Century German psychoanalyst.

To be sure, today's physicians have a sharply different method and objective than their profession's earliest practitioners. Many of the early medicine men strived to determine what actions by an individual had angered the gods or spirits, negative developments that motivated those entities to inflict their patients with pain or disease. Depending on the specific culture, potential treatments or perceived possible cures ranged from ritualistic dancing or chanting to direct methods such as touching.

Early Cultures Began Using Plants and Herbs

Historians tell us that many pre-historic cultures, particularly in North America, gradually began using specific plants and herbs to treat ailments or perceived problems that included sore throats, constipation, sleeplessness, and pain relievers. Many of these early remedies became the basis for herbs and human-produced drugs widely prescribed by modern medical professionals. Among the early medical success of pre-historic people:

- Herbs and minerals: Developed or identified herbs or other substances, deemed effective in the treatments of specific types of medical complaints.
- Trial and error: At least partly mirroring modern scientists efforts to undergo rigorous testing in the research and

- development process, pre-historic cultures pinpointed which substances worked and which failed at addressing specific ailments.

- Long-term efforts: Early cultures realized that many of the worst diseases or illnesses only hit an individual once—never returning again after immunity developed. For this reason, some people within specific pre-historic cultures apparently strived to suffer from mild cases of specific illnesses in order to prevent becoming extremely sick in the future.

Despite these initial strides, anthropologists urge us to remain cognizant that many of these early efforts lacked a rock-solid, scientific basis. For the most part, early medicine men were merely embracing or practicing the spiritual belief systems and traditions passed from generation to generation within their own cultures.

"People should think things out fresh and not just accept conventional terms and the conventional way of doing things," said R. Buckminster Fuller, a 20th Century American author, engineer and futurist.

Medicines Emerged as Life Expectancies Increased

At least according to numerous published accounts, average life expectancies many hundreds or thousands of years ago were only 25 to 40 years. That's a sharp contrast to a 75-to-81-year life span for today's newborns in the United States.

Scientists give vastly diverging theories on why the average lifespan has dramatically increased. They cite everything from improved nutrition to better overall housing. Yet, there's little denying that as life expectancies crept upward, the production, distribution and use of specified pharmaceuticals and herbs has steadily increased to significant levels.

Add to this the fact that early cultures lacked the modern machinery that improved and brought increased efficiency to the moving of heavy objects. Thousands or hundreds of years ago, many laborers were subjected to rigorous and potentially harmful lifting, sometimes causing extreme damage to their muscular structures and bones.

These jobs occasionally aggravated an extremely painful fracture-prone medical conditions such as rickets, the softening and deformation of bones, or osteomalacia, a milder adult form of the disease associated with a Vitamin D deficiency associated with a poor diet or a lack of adequate sunlight.

Meantime, as people made increasingly effective tools, improved farming methods and began constructing cities and towns, most cultures could only use any available possible pain-killing herbs that happened to grow in regions where they lived. This reigned as a sharply different process than today, when large distributors and pharmaceutical companies quickly identify and transport useful herbs and plants worldwide.

"Any sufficiently advanced technology is indistinguishable from magic," said Arthur C. Clark, a prolific and widely popular British science fiction writer in the 1900s and early 2000s.

The Use of Herbs and Pharmaceutical Medicines Spread

Historians admit they remain unsure as to precisely which specific herbs and plant remedies were used in many pre-historic cultures, at least judging by various published accounts of this intriguing topic.

Nonetheless, it remains clear that many people suffering from severe pains within diverse cultures thousands of years ago demanded, pleaded for or sought the types of remedies that many of us take for granted today. Some researchers have even argued or at least suggested that pre-historic people even employed healing clays— or "medicinal clays"—for certain healing or medicinal qualities, mimicking remedies used by certain wild animals.

Anthropologists have reported finding signs of widespread use of medicinal clays among various ancient indigenous cultures including Mesopotamia. Researchers believe people externally applied these materials to the skin during certain activities, such as bathing at health spas or taking mud baths.

At least some aspects of these early pre-historic or ancient-period traditions continue even today, particularly within certain realms of alternative medicine. For the most part, such treatments or applications are not recognized by practitioners of today's "standard, mainstream medicine" as having medically viable or therapeutic qualities.

Scientists and practitioners of homeopathic medicine outside the culture of mainstream physicians sometimes refer to the use of clays for medicinal purposes as "geophagy." Even the famous ancient

Greek physician and philosopher Galen noticed that certain wild animals including reptiles, birds and mammals sometime use clay to treat their illnesses or injuries. Historians have documented the increasingly widespread use of clays up to the present, from the medieval era through the Renaissance and beyond.

While many mainstream physicians argue otherwise, numerous homeopaths and practitioners of alternative medicine insist that some medicinal clays possess indisputable antibacterial qualities, making these materials effective in the treatment of surface pains.

According to an article in the "Journal of antimicroborial chemotherapy," certain iron-rich clays have been effective in killing some bacteria within test tubes. And, a 2008 article entitled "Healing Clays," stated that at least 20 of these bentonite-type materials showed promising results in fighting the "super-bug" bacterium MRSA—scientifically called "Methicillin-resistant Staphylococcus aureus."

As controversy continues to erupt as to the effectiveness of medicinal clays first used thousands of years ago, therapeutic mud baths remain increasingly popular within many cultures. And some mainstream medical facilities have experimented with the use of such substances at least in part for the treatment of war wounds. A 2008 article on Wired Dot Com noted that chemists had infused gauze with nano-particles of clay, drastically improving the ability to curtail blood loss.

These are just some examples of why scientists and physicians determined to whip the ravages of pain should continue researching and possibly implementing potential medical treatments first used long ago by pre-historic people.

Serious Pain Medicines and Physicians Emerged 4,000 Years Ago

Serious studies and efforts to address pain and ailments began about 2,000 years before Christ in the Egyptian, Mesopotamian and Babylonian cultures, according to various archeological reports and scientific documents. For the most part many medical advances and strategies in these regions avoided mysticism or citing the gods as reasons for painful ailments, but instead focused on potential scientific causes.

Particularly in the early Babylonian culture, physicians gradually began the process of diagnosing specific illnesses. These early doctors conducted physical examinations, before stating the prognosis or projected outcomes of specific individual patients. Along with the advent of issuing prescriptions, all these basic steps gradually emerged worldwide as the foundations and basic standards for today's general medical practices for fighting pain.

And, according to various quotations from the Bible's early sections, around 1,000 years before Christ the Hebrews realized the vital interaction between cleanliness and the prospects for good, pain-free health. For anyone suffering pain today, those early findings and advances in cultural changes established the necessary foundation for the ongoing need to keep materials free of germs and away from potentially harmful bacteria to lessen the probability of infections.

That age-old saying that "cleanliness is next to godliness," still holds true more than ever before—especially in matters involving the effective elimination, prevention and eradication of pain or the primary medical conditions that ignite such sensations.

"Keep your spirits up and your physical body as clean as possible," I tell many of my patients today, even some cancer patients or those treated for a wide variety of other ailments. "Besides good nutrition, a steady exercise regimen and adequate periods for sleep, keeping the body's surface free of potential infectious-causing viruses can go a long way in helping you to achieve and to maintain overall good, pain-free health."

Chapter 24

Early Alternative Medicine Also Emerged to Fight Pain

W hile the early foundations of today's mainstream standard medical practice evolved in Europe and the Middle East, early precursors of modern alternative treatments evolved in vastly different regions of the world such as China.

Within the Chinese culture, the prescribing of herbs and various natural plant-based substances for pain and illness is considered "mainstream." But for many people in the Western culture, particularly in the United States, such treatments are viewed as "alternative." Most such pain-fighting efforts that evolved in the Chinese culture, such as herbs and acupuncture, are never recognized by standard allopathic physicians in the U.S., where giant for-profit pharmaceutical companies rule the marketplace.

Sadly, from my view and from the perspective of many other American homeopaths, the basic culture of the USA ignores and even shuns the remarkable treatments first developed in China and other non-European countries thousands of years ago.

Perhaps this aspect—the occasional use of vital, pain-killing or health-enhancing herbs through my medical practice—angers or upsets at least some standard medical practitioners within our culture. In a sense, from their view, my treatment methods have rocked the proverbial apple cart. Is it possible that mainstream physicians feel threatened, as people from all over the world flock to my medical clinic in the Western United States?

Remember that while striving to fight and eliminate the pain and other ailments that my patients experience, as an integrative practitioner of medicine I sometimes use or prescribe herbal treatments or natural pain remedies that have proven effective for thousands of years within other cultures such as China.

"Here in America, we descended in blood and in spirit from revolutionists and rebels—men and women who dare to dissent from accepted doctrine," said Dwight David "Ike" Eisenhower, the 34th President of the United States and a five-star general in World War II. "As their heirs, may we never confuse honest dissent with disloyal subversion."

Early Chinese Medicines Can Help Fight Pain

Although many of today's mainstream American medical professionals might tell you otherwise, some of the various herbs, acupuncture methods and massages developed in early China can play a significant role in fighting pain.

Some critics argue that Chinese-based treatments ignore standard and acceptable scientific medical criteria. Perhaps such criticism stems at least in part from the fact that traditional Chinese medicine views the interconnection among the body's various organs at least partly on the basis of certain metaphysical principles. This emerges as a sharp contrast from mainstream medicines in our Western culture, where science-based medicine prevails—hinged largely on specific research involving specific bodily fuctions.

By contrast, since emerging thousands of years ago, basic medical practices embraced by the Chinese culture blame illness on an imbalance among the body's various sections and functional organs.

As you might imagine, some mainstream traditional doctors in our Western culture whine like little babies when they see that growing numbers of patients worldwide agree with my analysis in this regard. To these upset doctors, I have to say that "why should we ignore and refuse to recognize effective treatments that a vast majority of the world's people use and fully accept? And, just because an overall standard allopathic treatment method is developed in the United States—hooked largely to big pharmaceutical companies— why should those systems be considered better in every instance, relegated as the only viable options?"

Generally, the practitioners of Chinese medicines strive to use everything from herbs and minerals to animal products and acupuncture in treating particular inter-related organ systems. Many of the harshest critics are quick to say that such treatments lack any verifiable and quantifiable scientific basis, while producing questionable results.

Such critics undoubtedly cringe at video presentations on my Web site, DrForsythe.com. These heart-felt, compelling and magnetic proclamations come from steadily growing numbers of my patients from around the world. Some of these emotional statements feature patients who had once lost hope for physical improvements, before my treatments left them pain-free or at least feeling less pain and suffering.

Standard Physicians Tell You These Methods are "Far-Fetched"

Perhaps worried or fearful that the integrative medical practices such as mine will endanger their livelihoods, today's doctors within our mainstream American culture eagerly strive to label practitioners such as me as "quacks" or "mavericks."

Maybe this stems at least partly from the fact that pain and illness treatments that homeopaths recommend sometimes include non-traditional methods such as message, breathing and meditation exercises—or any of a wide variety of other methods seen as "off-the-wall" by mainstream physicians. Needless to say, today's "Big Pharma," the huge pharmaceutical conglomerates and standard-medicine doctors in the U.S. culture worry that they'll miss out on the big bucks if patients know they can go elsewhere.

The list of herbs, meditation styles and acupuncture treatments—all proven as consistently effective in the treatments of pain—is seemingly endless. And, of course, in the meantime many of the specific drugs and treatments embraced and commonly used in the mainstream U.S. medical industry also have proven effective as well. But many of these mainstream medications are riddled with severe and potentially fatal side effects.

While keeping the best, most effective medical methods from both cultures at the forefront, physicians such as me who fully understand, prescribe and embrace both systems have an opportunity to teach the general public. Personally, I feel obligated to educate patients worldwide that both medical systems have important roles in providing vital and necessary care to people who depend on our expertise.

Through the coming years, as society enjoys the continual new and improved advancements in medical technology, homeopaths and standard physicians must do more to appreciate and embrace each others' specific and general treatment methods.

From my view, in an ideal world, as we strive to battle the physical and emotional pains that plague our patients, physicians have an obligation to take essential, urgent and progressive strides in working for the betterment of the people we help. A key part of this process should entail the melding of the alternative homeopathic medicines and so-called mainstream medical practices.

Ideally, practitioners of these systems should meld their clinics, centralized in the same facilities. Such goals strike me and many other doctors as logical and even necessary for the betterment of patients. After all, standard allopathic physicians and homeopaths have already melded or integrated their practices in many other parts of the world including much of Europe and Asia.

Yet at least for the present, such overall efforts seem almost unmentionable within most of today's mainstream American culture. This leads me and the handful of other integrative physicians to openly pose such questions as, "If other areas of the world are benefiting patients by bringing together these medical systems, why should we be prevented from doing the same?"

Nations Other Than China Also Contributed to Alternative Medicines

As controversy continues to erupt about the effectiveness of homeopathic medicine, we need to remain cognizant that a wide variety of other cultures besides the Chinese also made significant contributions to today's alternative treatment systems.

The various cultures, nations and continents where natural plant-based remedies evolved during the past 2,000 years include the Germanic region, the vast areas of Central America and South America and across much of Africa as well. Through trial and error, various cultures that followed the pre-historic era found or rediscovered essential plants and minerals that are often prescribed today by homeopaths for pain treatments.

Through the Middle Ages between the fifth century after Christ and the 1400s, primary regions including the weakening Western Roman and Eastern Roman empires strived to identify and develop treatments for various painful and sometimes fatal illnesses. Historians tell us that during this period as a crossroads between the east and the west Persia served as an integral site during the developments of ancient Indian and Greek medicines.

As the Islamic civilization grew and prospered, Arab physicians played integral roles in developing vital and essential medical systems. These ranged from surgeries to pharmacies and the development of various pharmaceutical products including some for the treatment of pain.

Meantime, during the same 1,000-year span, gradually as the authority of the former Roman Empire disintegrated, Christian-based societies and cultures began independently developing, embracing or formalizing the medical infrastructure. While hospitals started emerging, some medical professionals began to drop the ancient teachings of the Romans and Greeks on how to treat pain—and instead commenced the development of new and unique treatments, often based on their own observations.

Rapid and essential advancements followed through the Renaissance from the 14th through the 17th centuries, when a cultural movement embraced the development of the arts and the sciences throughout most of Europe. At an increasingly rapid pace during this period, physicians and scientists began examining the bodies of living people, dissected cadavers and launched a vast array of experiments.

Essentially, all this was done in large part in an effort to determine the causes of the body's various physical pains, how those signals were identified, transmitted to and interpreted by the brain, and possible ways of treating or eliminating such sensations.

Although science had made tremendous strides in these efforts, extremely painful conditions such as arthritis persisted while possible remedies remained fairly limited just 500 years ago.

Chapter 25

Wars Enabled People to Learn About Pain

Whether we like to admit this or not, throughout history and especially during the last 300 years the world's bloodiest wars played a pivotal role in enabling physicians to learn more about the phenomena of pain and to develop effective treatments.

"Doctors will have more lives to answer for in the next world than even we generals," said Napoleon Bonaparte, the French emperor and military leader during the late 1700s and early 1800s. Particularly from the Renaissance through the present day, as the weapons employed in wars became increasingly sophisticated and battle zones stretched for thousands of miles, physicians were forced to treat everything from wounds to extreme hunger and diseases such as dysentery on a massive scale.

Man's so-called "inhumanity to man" had spread and intensified painful conditions, in many cases impacting tens of millions of people. Such horrid conditions played an integral role in forcing medical advancements in the treatment of pain and disease that persist even today, benefiting people in eras and regions of peace.

Of course, many wars throughout history have ravaged and decimated vast cultures. But the intensity, number and ferocity of such conflicts intensified in the 1700s. The Great Northern War stretching from 1700 to 1721 started this era of seemingly non-stop death and destruction involving 13 countries or empires from Great Britain to the Ottoman Empire. This marked just the start of the horrors that were to plague that era; historians tell us that at least 70 wars erupted worldwide during the 1700s, including the American Revolutionary War from 1775 to 1783.

Lacking the fast-paced medical technology prevalent on today's battlefields, during those clashes tens of thousands—and collectively perhaps millions—of soldiers suffered horrifically painful wounds. Many of them were left mortally wounded on battlefields, stricken by wretched and hellish pains. Lots of these victims spent their final minutes, hours or even days, wailing for help or relief from pain that never subsided until unconsciousness and eventual death, which many of them apparently welcomed after intense suffering.

Civil War Advancements Helped Alleviate Pain

Physicians from the Union and Confederate armies made tremendous gains during the American Civil War from 1961 to 1865, during which an estimated 260,000 soldiers died and perhaps tens of thousands suffered the loss of limbs. Huge casualty totals in many bloody battles forced physicians to devise methods of quickly alleviating extreme pain, enabling doctors or medical crews to administer life-saving battlefield amputations. Some basic techniques these physicians devised emerged as the forefront of primary pain-fighting strategies employed today in both war and peacetime environments.

"It is well that war is so terrible, lest we grow fond of it," said Gen. Robert E. Lee, commander of the Confederate Army of Northern Virginia.

Historians tell us that wars elsewhere before this great American confrontation mostly featured relatively small armies, primarily due to the logistical challenges of amassing troops, plus the difficulties of generating efficient supply lines. And, prior to the Civil War, notoriously inaccurate musket fire kept casualties to a minimum.

Those trends took a sharp reversal during the American confrontation as trains, supply lines and new telegraph systems increased efficiency. Adding to the misery, the advent of mass-produced canned foods and vastly more efficient Minié ball weaponry enabled massive numbers of troops to essentially become efficient killing machines in high numbers in confined areas.

Within months after the war began, the Union Army began requiring that each regiment recruit at least one surgeon and one assistant surgeon. When mobile medical transportation systems proved inefficient as thousands of soldiers died, the military developed an all-new ambulance corps in order to accelerate transportation of the pain-stricken, wounded soldiers to hospitals. Although relatively crude by today's standards, these systems emerged as to the early precursors to today's modern ambulance systems. Even then doctors realized the urgency of getting patients treatment as soon as possible in order to treat pain, injury, illness and hemorrhaging.

Battling Physical and Emotional Pains Became a Top Priority

The steadily increasing magnitude and intensity of the war forced the Union to upgrade transportation, hospitals, nursing crews and in-the-field educational procedures by early 1863. Meantime, the Confederates' medical core was organized much faster but it lacked the non-stop supply of vital and essential pain-killers and surgeons available in the north. Within the war's first few years, some Confederate troops were forced to seize buildings for use as temporary hospitals.

On both sides, for the first time in the history of war soldiers and their industrial supporters strived to amass extensive non-stop quantities of alcohol and the organic compound of chloroform in an effort to alleviate pains suffered by the continually swelling numbers of severely wounded.

Much of the time during amputations, the patients remained at least somewhat awake while never realizing much of the resulting pain, at least according to some published accounts. From the standpoint of today's physicians such as I, these developments—although relatively crude and non-sophisticated in nature—marked a significant development in the treatment of sudden, intense and debilitating pain.

Stewart Brand, an American writer best known as editor of the "Whole Earth Catalogue," has been quoted as saying that "Once a new technology rolls over you, if you're not part of the steamroller, you're part of the road." Sure enough, historians tell us that these new or upgraded pain-killing methods on a massive scale forced battlefield physicians to intensify and continually improve their pain fighting methods.

In the form of a sweet-smelling condensed liquid, chloroform soon gained a well-deserved reputation as extremely dangerous. Derived primarily from naturally occurring ocean-based substances such as seaweed, chloroform started gaining popularity as an anesthetic in 1847, just 14 years before the Civil War erupted.

According to some historical accounts, chloroform's earliest use as an anesthetic emerged when a Scottish physician, James Young Simpson, began administering the substance to women undergoing childbirth. The popularity of using this substance soon spread as increasing numbers of physicians realized chloroform's ability to suppress the central nervous mechanism, the body's system of communicating pain signals from the site of a wound to the brain.

Pain-Killing Drugs Began Growing at a Rapid Pace As Wars Spread

By the time the Civil War began some U.S. surgeons and general physicians had already started using chloroform at an increasingly rapid pace. The war quickly brought chloroform to the forefront, as the general public began perceiving the substance as a crucial tool in fighting or warding off pain, especially during amputations or extensive surgeries.

The widespread popularity of chloroform soon took a sharp downswing, especially during the initial decades after the war. Physicians and their patients gradually began to realize and acknowledge chloroform's toxicity, which sometimes caused what some people hailed as "sudden sniffer's death," commonly known today as sudden cardiac arrhythmia.

Through much of the mid-1800s chloroform emerged as a preferred anesthetic, temporarily exceeding the popularity of ether. But ether re-emerged as a predominant favorite by the early 20th Century as physicians began avoiding the use of chloroform.

The Ether Pain Killer Swelled in Popularity

From the 1200s through the 1500s, scientists, researchers and physicians began to realize and appreciate the pain-killing attributes of ether, a colorless and highly flammable liquid created when distilling a mixture of sulfuric acid and ethanol. During that period, doctors began to realize ether's indisputable qualities as an "analgesic," the term used in designating any specific drug as a painkiller.

Although ether had remained well known among scientists for several centuries, like chloroform had this substance emerged into the widespread public scene in the 1840s. Early in that decade, the physician Crawford Williamson Long demonstrated in private sessions the use of ether as a general anesthetic. Soon afterward, in Boston, Mass, in October 1846, William T.G. Morton gave a public demonstration of the use of ether as a general anesthetic.

Even today, at least judging by some news accounts, ether hails as a preferred choice as a general anesthetic in some developing nations where the substance remains readily available thanks to its relatively low cost when compared to the most popular drugs in its class. However, like many other powerful pharmaceutical products that target pain, ether became a "recreational drug" that some people abused because of its impact on the central nervous system.

An ancient Chinese proverb proclaims that "it is easy to get a thousand prescriptions, but hard to get one single remedy." Indeed, especially during the late 1800s, people began devising, producing or distributing various types of analgesics at a rapidly increasing rate, even some substances that had been known for thousands of years but that had received little overall publicity until then. As a result, society began to recognize and even ban or discourage some substances due to their negative side effects.

Some greedy companies and individual consumers eager to profit from or to abuse painkillers devised crafty methods of distributing and consuming such substances, particularly during the late 1800s. Some researchers claim certain cough drops during this period contained both ether and alcohol. Many of the most ardent consumers of these products reportedly were women, perhaps— some researchers believed—because adult females were often banned or discouraged from attending social events where men enjoyed alcohol.

In John Irving's novel, "The Cider House Rules," which later became a 1999 Academy Award®-winning movie by the same name, the character Dr. Wilbur Larch portrayed by Michael Caine in the film, succumbs to an addiction to ether consumption. The fictional doctor dies at the beginning of the 20th Century at an orphanage. This award-winning book and film epitomized the social views of the early 20th Century, when some emerging analgesics became vilified and shunned almost as quickly as they had surged in popularity.

Chapter 26

Pain-Killing Aspirin Emerged onto the Scene

The generic, prevalent and often-effective substance we commonly call aspirin has been known to scientists since the antiquity period several hundred years after Christ. Yet, amazingly, the vital, much-appreciated substance was not widely distributed and used until 1899 on the heels of the Spanish-American War the previous two years.

At seemingly the speed of light this so-called "wonder drug" engulfed the medical industry, while satisfying the urgent needs of individual consumers seeking relief from persistent and nagging aches and pains. By 1910, as the Industrial Revolution clicked into full gear, aspirin emerged as a common, accepted and expected feature of the American culture.

"Wine and cheese are like ageless companions, like aspirin and aches, or June and moon, or good people and noble virtues," said Mary Francis Kennedy Fisher, a widely acclaimed and respected 20th Century author.

Although scientists had known the many benefits of aspirin comprised of willow bark extract for more than 1,000 years, it wasn't until the mid-1800s that physicians began to fully appreciate and disseminate news of this substance's many wonderful qualities—particularly the ability to alleviate or eliminate pain, lessen fevers and relieve swelling.

Some historians believe that from 1803 to 1806 the widely acclaimed explorers Meriwether Lewis and William Clark used willow bark extract to treat fevers in their famous exploration of western North America. From the mid- to late-1800s scientists experimented with and prescribed specific chemicals known as the active ingredients of willow bark. This research culminated in 1897, when the drug and dye firm Bayer™ worked with many of these researchers in devising methods of generating the active ingredients of the willow bark extracts.

The massive social change evolved in 1899 when Bayer™ dubbed the resulting substance "aspirin." At the time the word was a brand name of the Bayer™ company, but the firm lost exclusive rights to produce and distribute the drug in numerous countries. Amid the same generation, within 20 years in 1918 the popularity of aspirin skyrocketed when this amazing substance proved effective in relieving or at least addressing some symptoms during the worldwide flu pandemic that killed millions of people.

Aspirin Became a Basic, Integral Tool in Battling Pain

Even today, scientists and amazed physicians are discovering and appreciating the many stupendous benefits that aspirin can offer. Key among these is the ability to thin the blood, reducing the likelihood of death if taken at the onset of heart attacks. Some physicians swear to the irrefutable benefits of using typical aspirin as an anti-clotting agent, often effective as a preventative measure in battling cardiac problems and strokes.

All along, many of the world's largest, most greedy pharmaceutical companies undoubtedly dislike aspirin because it's relatively cheap for consumers and can easily be purchased at most pharmacies, grocery stores and convenience stores without prescriptions from physicians.

Thus, consumers seeking relief from basic pains or aches often can sidestep expensive visits to doctors' offices. As a result, Big Pharma misses out on at least some potential opportunities to gouge the public, the way these huge pharmaceutical companies do when charging $5 or much more for individual pain-killing pills other than aspirin.

All along, despite its many positive potential benefits, aspirin poses at least some possible drawbacks. The primary disadvantage occurs when aspirin causes or sets the stage for stomach upsets or ulcers, especially when taken if the person fails to eat immediately before or while ingesting these pills.

Aspirin also gets little or no attention from some people suffering from intense pains because this generic product is much less powerful than many highly addictive substances. Still, aspirin remains a shining star within the realm of analgesics for the very reason that it's non-addictive on a physiological level. Of course, some people might take too much aspirin in an effort to satisfy their apparent psychological needs, but overall such problems seem rare and much less harmful than full-fledged pain-killing narcotics.

Aspirin's Role Remains Controversial ~ Although Generic

Even during the advent of the 21st Century more than 100 years after the widespread emergence of aspirin historians remain at conflict as to which scientists played the most significant roles in contributing the Bayer™ company's efforts. Still, there is no denying that aspirin has played—and will continue to play—a significant and essential role in medicine.

This holds true even though numerous other over-the-counter or non-prescription pain-killers emerged for general purchases by consumers in the mid-1900s. These include acetaminophen introduced in 1956 and Ibuprofen launched just six years later, both listed as generally safe, low-power drugs with little harmful side effects when taken at suggested doses.

These developments gave generic aspirin a run for its money, so to speak, during a period when some observers contend the overall popularity of the willow bark extract finally began to wane. Ever since then, scientists and particularly the research and development divisions of huge pharmaceutical companies have worked non-stop in efforts to discover or create new, effective low-range pain killers on the level of aspirin.

The emergence of acetaminophen and Ibuprofen came in a vastly different era of professionally acceptable marketing and promotions within the medical industry. During the years immediately after the official launch of aspirin, a vast array of medical professionals from doctors to hospital operators received packets of aspirin from Bayer™—encouraging them to publish research papers on this drug.

When doctors began documenting and reporting positive results, Bayer™ continued efforts to patent and trademarks for aspirin. These efforts proved fruitless, however, because numerous companies had already begun producing and distributing aspirin by the time World War I erupted in 1914.

Even today, the specific ways that the various chemicals within aspirin actually generate positive symptoms remains in dispute. At first, some researchers and original developers of aspirin claimed that the willow tree bark derivative somehow blocked the transmission of pain signals from the nervous system to the brain. However, according to one published report, at least one researcher who used animals in tests concluded that aspirin's chemical compounds worked at the actual source of pain, such as a wound. While scientists continue to argue the specific reasons for aspirin's fantastic qualities, this low-cost drug will likely remain an essential tool in the pain-fighting analgesic category for many years.

Chapter 27

Intravenous Therapy or IVs Drastically Improved Delivery

Perhaps one of the greatest, most essential medical innovations that clicked into gear as the Industrial Revolution reached full steam was intravenous therapy—commonly known as "IVs." At a steadily increasing pace starting in the late 1800s, these devices were used for a variety of methods of delivering vital fluids, drugs and eventually plasma to wounded or ill patients.

IV devices entail the use of hypodermic needles or thin catheters, inserted into the patient's veins for the disbursement of vital, life-saving fluids, pharmaceuticals or even blood transfusions. For cases involving pain, intravenous devices give medical professionals and doctors the ability to quickly administer essential drugs or substances, particularly in life-threatening situations.

The use of IVs for specific uses from drug infusions to transfusions came in various phases through the 20th Century. From the start, the devices played essential roles in alleviating the pains and symptoms of dehydration, quickly re-hydrating the body following the extreme and life-threatening loss of essential fluids.

Just like doctors had done with aspirin, the medical industry quickly accepted the IV as an essential treatment tool. Physicians systematically in phases accepted new and essential uses for intravenous therapy. This all became possible thanks to drip chambers that prevented air from entering the body's blood circulation systems.

As the 20th Century genius Albert Einstein once proclaimed, "It has become appallingly obvious that our technology has exceeded our humanity." Surely there could be no denying that throughout that century people began murdering other humans at a previously unheard of, horrendous and horrific rate. Seemingly with each new wave of killings, however, from the various wars and massacres throughout that era science continually developed and improved new essential pain-killing devices like IVs.

Just like all other primary pharmaceuticals and medical devices, the IV units posed potential setbacks or complications to patients. Possible negative risks ranged from painful infection and phlebitis or swelling caused by such conditions. Other potential dangers from intravenous therapy include: fluid overload, putting excessive amounts of fluids into the body faster than it can absorb; hypothermia, when the body absorbs excessive levels of cold fluids; imbalances in the body's chemical levels or electrolytes; and potentially fatal embolisms, caused by delivery of blood clots, air bubbles or other solids.

While all these possible hazards are indeed serious, the countless benefits of intravenous therapy far outweigh the risks. In fact, during the first decade of my career in the 1970s as a full-time oncologist, I personally administered many chemotherapy treatments via IV to my cancer patients. Much of these laborious and complex chores needed my full attention, since my personal staff and hospital personnel levels lacked adequate numbers of certified, trained nurses or other medical professionals to handle all of those chores.

James W. Forsythe, M.D., H.M.D.

Wars Played a Pivotal Role in the Fight Against Pain

As we've already seen, wars played a pivotal role in generating essential medical innovations in the fight against pain. The USA's military has been fully cognizant of these important and necessary developments, motivated to launch the U.S. Army Medical Museum—which later became the National Museum of Health and Medicine.

Located in Washington, D.C., the facility was launched in 1862 at the beginning of the Civil War. Military leaders and physicians realized the essential need to accumulate and study biological specimens to advance the knowledge of doctors and wound treatment. Researchers and museum officials began accumulating bits or fragments of weaponry from battles, plus parts of human bodies treated for war wounds.

The museum's many unique and compelling displays or holdings of more than 25 million artifacts include—most famously—pieces of President Abraham Lincoln's skull; the Derringer used by his assassin, John Wilkes Booth; a probe used to locate the bullet; and a portion of an autopsy surgeon's shirt stained with Lincoln's blood. Streams of people visit the museum yearly, many of them extremely curious about almost anything that involved the infliction, suffering and treatment of intense pain.

Thankfully, our nation's military leaders continued these vital efforts of amassing artifacts and essential medical information during subsequent wars, all major military conflicts of the 20th Century. Medications developed independent of the military such as aspirin and the growing use of IVs were deployed to treat pain and wounds in World War I, World War II, the Korean War, the Vietnam War, the battle of Granada, and the first Gulf War in the early 1990s.

Many pain-killing pharmaceuticals that consumers use today were initially administered at or during these conflicts. Especially in Vietnam in the 1960s and early 1970s, the military developed and honed the use of quickly delivering wounded soldiers via helicopter from battle zones to medical facilities or hospitals. Similar patient-delivery systems soon carried over into civilian life throughout the USA, enabling physicians to quickly treat pain, wounds or extreme illnesses such as heart attacks or strokes.

Chapter 28

Addictive Morphine Entered Battlefields and General Medicine

Thanks largely to the increasingly common use of hypodermic needles and IVs, the extremely potent opiate morphine began making its way into battlefields to save wounded U.S. soldiers from the ravages of pain—particularly during the Vietnam War. The hypodermic needle, highly effective for the injection of drugs into the body, was actually invented in the 1850s, the same decade when several other significant medical advances emerged in the years immediately before the Civil War.

Although initially used primarily by medical professionals, hypodermic needles were so specialized and easy to use that some drug addicts eventually became adept at administering their own hits. Like morphine, during the 1900s the hypodermic needle emerged as a double-edged sword, essential in the legitimate and necessary administering of medical treatments, and for the extremely harmful use by addicts as well. Composed of pointed, hallowed-out stainless steel tubes, hypodermic syringes became just as important to heroin addicts as to diabetics who needed to inject their own insulin.

"It is the paradox of life that the way to miss pleasure is to seek it first," said Hugo Black, a 20th Century American jurist, lawyer and politician. "The very first condition of lasting happiness is that life should be full of purpose, aiming at something outside self."

Morphine gave many horribly injured U.S. soldiers just such a reason for hope, in many cases quickly blocking or masking painful sensations. Some physicians have even gone so far as to claim that morphine is the benchmark or a gold standard among analgesics, thanks to its ability to relieve patients from intense suffering and extreme pain. But like other opiates made from opium, such as the dreadful drug heroin, morphine targets the body's central nervous system.

Doctors will be among the first people to tell you that morphine is so intense and effective at blocking painful sensations that—although some individuals can tolerate the substance—other persons can quickly become psychologically addicted. The actual physiological or biology-based addictions can take much longer to kick into full gear, some researchers say.

After their tours of duty or upon being discharged following medical treatment, some Vietnam War veterans returned to U.S. society with debilitating addictions to morphine. For many, these additions progressed to heroin and other harmful narcotics. More than ever before, and at an increasingly intense pace, the many benefits and severe drawbacks of pain and of the increasing number of medications to hinder that sensation spilled over into the mainstream of popular American culture.

Morphine's Popularity Gradually Grew for More Than 2,000 Years

Long before the Vietnam War, as far back as the early Byzantine era 300 years after Christ, alchemists—specialists in transforming metals—began tinkering with efforts to create early forms of morphine. Following more than 1,200 years in the early 1500s the Austrian alchemist, botanist and physician Paracelsus wrote of a new highly potent pain killer, an early precursor of morphine, but recommended its use only on rare occasions.

According to "Molecular, clinical and environmental toxicology" published in 2009, the modern-day equivalent of morphine was discovered in 1804 by a German pharmacist, Friedrich Wilhelm Adam Sertürner. Historians credit this creative genius with being the first person to use opium in isolating the essential substances for morphine. By some accounts, Sertürner named this new creation after the Greek god Morpheus, hailed in mythology as "the god of dreams."

Thirteen years after Sertürner discovery, in 1817 a pharmaceutical company began distributing morphine as an analgesic that also could be used for treating alcoholism and even opium addictions. Sales increased in both volume and geographic area through the next several decades. However, by the time the Civil War erupted in the early 1860s scientists had begun to acknowledge that morphine was highly addictive.

"All sin tends to be addictive, and the terminal point of addiction is what is called damnation," said Wystan Hugh Auden, an early 20th

Century English-born American dramatist, poet and editor. Indeed, according to some published accounts, an arguably high estimate of 400,000 Civil War soldiers became addicted to morphine. Although such totals seem highly questionable by some accounts, there seems to be little doubt that morphine took a heavy toll on American society a century before the Vietnam War.

In fact, Bayer™, the same company instrumental in initially launching and distributing aspirin in the late 19th Century, launched the widespread production and distribution of heroin in 1898, just 24 years after synthesizing that substance from morphine. Heroin got plenty of attention, hailed as about 2 ½ times more powerful than morphine and possessing an impressive capability of moving more easily from the blood to the brain.

Powerful Painkillers Became Illegal

The extreme addictiveness coupled with the mega-powerful potency of morphine motivated U.S. lawmakers to make possession of this substance illegal nationwide. With passage in 1914 of the Harrison Narcotics Tax Act, Congress outlawed this opiate-based substance unless accompanied by a prescription from a licensed physician. The law marked a significant social change—the banning of a powerful substance that much of the public yearned for, wanted and needed largely to fight pain. The very substances that people craved to fight extremely uncomfortable sensations became illegal unless used under medical supervision, and for a very good reason.

Thus, at the same time that technology advanced society's ability to discover, produce and distribute mass quantities of pain killers, people in many segments of the entire U.S. society experienced and suffered from the many negative side effects of narcotics. Besides opium-based products, the Harrison Narcotics Act imposed stiff restrictions on the production, distribution and possession of substances derived from cocoa leaves—the key ingredient in the highly addictive narcotic cocaine and once a primary ingredient in the earliest version of the popular soda, Coca-Cola™.

Morphine, opium and heroin reigned as the most powerful and most frequently prescribed top-level, analgesic-class narcotic pain killers through most of the early 1900s. Just like aspirin had, morphine remained on the market for many years before physicians began to realize and understand how its primary ingredients interact with the body. Meantime, scientists strived to understand and identify key factors that make morphine effective.

Amazingly, according to a 2005 article "Human white blood cells synthesize morphine," scientists discovered that a specific receptor within the human body reacts only to this narcotic.

When used as an analgesic, doctors use morphine to relieve pain in certain types of medical conditions. The primary or most prevalent conditions are for:

- Myocardial infractions: Most commonly known as "heart attacks," these occur when the blood supply to the heart gets interrupted, resulting in an extremely painful condition.

- Sickle-cell crisis: These conditions caused by a blood disorder sometimes result in extreme pain, when certain cells lose flexibility and thereby generate complications.

- Extreme conditions: These pains occur as a result of everything from trauma caused by car wrecks and war wounds to conditions resulting from surgery.

- Chronic pain: This long-term or persistent condition results from such relentless debilitating conditions as cancer, kidney stones or severe muscular-skeletal injuries or diseases.

Morphine is also sometimes used for a variety of other conditions, sometimes in consortium with other drugs, for everything from severe coughs to an adjunct to general anesthesia and even for a chronic diarrhea associated with AIDS.

This drug is most often administered via IV, but other methods include orally, via injection, or inhaling—a method commonly used by abusers. Even when used in antibacterial-free medical environments, morphine can result in serious medical complications such as addiction, constipation, and the unintentional transmission of harmful viruses in instances where blood or other substances are not adequately checked beforehand.

Although a potentially dangerous and highly addictive narcotic, morphine can serve a legitimate and often-necessary role in the world's non-stop battle against physical pain. In my personal and professional view, this often misunderstood substance should remain available as a vital potential tool in the medical industry's battle to give patients relief and thereby opening a pathway for potential recovery.

James W. Forsythe, M.D., H.M.D.

Opium Pain-Killers Were Used For Thousands of Years

The so-called big brother or master of morphine is the naturally growing and highly dangerous substance opium. Highly addictive, this plant used since the Stone Age and eventually by such societies as the early Romans also was used extensively and got introduced to the general public during the American Civil War of the 1860s.

Used as the primary ingredient for the deadly and highly addictive heroin, opium is so powerful that just 12 percent of it contains the primary effective ingredients of morphine. More than 500 years ago the Chinese recognized opium's tremendous power, as various segments of that society began adopting the drug for recreational use.

"Among the remedies which it has pleased Almighty God to give man to relieve his sufferings, none is so universal and so efficacious as opium," said Thomas Sydenham, a 17th Century English physician. Such observations may have hit the proverbial bull's-eye dead center from the medical aspect, yet there can be no denying that opium has generated various sufferings throughout humanity, from severe addictions, to wrecked personal finances and broken families. Once again, with opium we realize the need to acknowledge the fact that the best, most effective pain killers also can create great harm.

"Nobody will laugh long who deals much with opium; its pleasures even are of a grave and solemn complexion," said Thomas de Quincey, a 19th Century English author and intellectual who wrote "Confessions of an English Opium-Eater" in 1821.

The opium trade became such an important economic force for the British Empire that from 1839 to 1858 during the "Opium Wars" the Europeans strived to continue distribution of the substance in China despite its emperor's ban on such commerce. Opium poppies are grown and harvested predominantly in Southern Asia including vastly divergent nations like India and Afghanistan. Archaeologists also found evidence of opium use long ago in Spain, Switzerland and Germany, according to some published accounts.

Researchers say that the use, distribution and trade of opium became so prevalent more than 1,000 years ago that the drug spread into the early Greek, Mediterranean and European cultures. Eventually after opium was introduced to China, about 800 years after Christ within the Persian area of the Middle East some physicians began using opium to treat melancholy and as an anesthetic.

"Opium teaches only one thing, which is that aside from physical suffering, there is nothing real," said Andre Malreaux, an award-winning 20th Century author, statesman and French adventurer.

Opium Blasted into the Mainstream Culture

Opium had become such a mainstay within the European and eventually the American medical culture that—by some accounts—it was among substances used to treat U.S. President William Henry Harrison after he contracted a fatal bout of pneumonia amid inclement weather in March 1841. The ninth U.S. president, he became the first of our nation's chief executives to die in office, 32 days after his inauguration.

Some historians have claimed that opium treatments worsened Harrison's physical condition along with fruitless efforts to use leeches and castor oil. Despite such setbacks, according to a 2008 issue of the "American Journal of Pharmaceutical Education," during the Civil War the Union Army issued what—at least to me—seemed like a mind-boggling, staggering 500,000 opium pills, and 2.8 million ounces of opium tincture.

By today's medical standards, at least from my professional view, such widespread distribution of the drug was highly dangerous from a societal standpoint. Yet rather than sharply criticizing those efforts, we should remain cognizant that for the most part many physicians were merely administering what they considered the best-available pain remedies for their era.

"The expense of a war could be paid in time; but the expense of opium, when once the habit is formed, will only increase with time," said Townsend Harris, a New York merchant and a minor politician in the 1800s.

According to a 2008 article, "Drug Research and the Health of Women," between 66 percent and 75 percent of the 150,000-200,000 opiate addicts in the United States in the late 19th Century were women—most of whom received opium as a prescription for female-related medical situations such as menstrual pain.

During the final decades of the 19th Century American communities began recognizing the ravages of opium, placing legal restrictions on the drug in 1875 in San Francisco. By 1919, tough regulations spread throughout California and eventually nationwide.

Opium-based Pain Killers Reigned Supreme

Sadly, at least from the view of many physicians within the mainstream medical community, throughout the early 20th Century painkillers derived from opium or synthetic versions of that substance remained the most effective drugs for painkilling. This ignited and spread the overwhelming and extremely dangerous potential for life-changing addictions.

Even the advent of synthetic opiates failed to stem this tide, such as the 1937 introduction of methadone and fentanyl in the late 1950s. Despite these advancements or additions, the U.S. military's combat medics still preferred to carry morphine. Perhaps largely for this reason, morphine is still legally produced in various nations primarily in Asia and South America. Despite the U.S. involvement in a war against the Taliban in Afghanistan, that nation remains the world's top illegal producer of poppies for the eventual production of heroin smuggled to the United States and Europe.

Meantime, the demand for opium for legitimate medicinal reasons including the production of morphine became so intense that in 2006 a drug company received permission from Britain to legally harvest poppies in that region. In a sense the so-called battle between good and evil get intermixed and confused, since drug abusers and legitimate users of opiate-based pharmaceuticals continue to show strong worldwide demand.

Chapter 29

Many "Recreational Drugs" Are Also Effective Pain Killers

Lots of the world's most sought-after narcotics commonly referred to as "recreational drugs," also are the most powerful substances at fighting pain. Besides being used for legitimate medical reasons, some narcotics including certain pain killers are sometimes used for spiritual reasons or in an effort by athletes to improve their performance.

Once again, the many potential positive results offered by legitimate but highly addictive pain killers threaten much of society with potentially negative consequences. When getting legitimate prescriptions of pain-fighting medication at pharmacies, some patients see required and highly necessary warnings such as "avoid driving when using this medication," or "must eat with food when ingesting." When refusing to follow such guidelines, patients put themselves and others in serious jeopardy.

Besides opiates, this pain-killing category also includes salicylates, which—like aspirin—contain substances derived from willow tree bark. Besides the treatment of pain and swelling, these specific acids offer a wide range of possible uses, from applications for acne, warts and corns to the production of products such as shampoo.

Even these lower-level pain killers at the level of aspirin have negative side effects. Some research shows that the active ingredient salicylic acid from the willow tree bark can be a factor in hearing loss.

Compounding matters, numerous narcotics sometimes deemed "recreational drugs" often are used as tranquilizers, for the primary purpose of sedating a person during a painful medical procedure. The many substances in the tranquilizer category, lots of them helpful in the treatment or avoidance of pain or to address anxiety, include barbiturates, ethanol and a vast range of other potentially harmful substances.

As if all these weren't already enough to cause concern, a vast range of drugs are abused by recreational users as hallucinogens, the same substances also employed on occasion within the legitimate medical profession in the treatment of pain or psychological conditions.

These include drugs in the "psychedelic" category, a term first made popular in the common U.S. vernacular during the so-called "drug revolution" and "social revolution" of the 1960s. The phrase "turn on, tune in, drop out" swept through the American counterculture that decade, popularized by Timothy Leary, a psychologist who touted what he perceived as the emotional, therapeutic, spiritual and emotional benefits generated by psychedelic drugs.

From my view, and from the perspective of a vast majority of licensed physicians, the use of psychedelic drugs is no laughing matter, but instead an issue of serious importance. Anyone considering the use of such substances, even for the intended purpose of coping with the sensations of physical or emotional pain, should do so only under the recommendation, continuous observation and care of a certified doctor.

Medicinal Marijuana Complicates the Mix

The super-charged, highly emotional issue of whether marijuana should be used in treating pain and illness erupted across the American political landscape during the final decades of the 20th Century and though the first decade of the current era.

Needless to say, this issue steadily evolved into perhaps the most hotly debated choice involving the treatment of pain, taking much of the spotlight in the mainstream media. To say that "weed," "grass" or "smokes" are harmless sparks the ire of people who swear that such treatments are merely an excuse for getting high.

Advocates of such treatments, the people who argue that such systems should get legitimized worldwide, insist that smoking or eating marijuana is highly effective in the treatment of chemotherapy, AIDS, nausea, vomiting, anorexia, pain and other ailments.

"Who benefits from keeping marijuana illegal?" asked George Soros, a Hungarian-American financier, philanthropist and businessman. "The greatest beneficiaries are the criminal organizations in Mexico, and elsewhere that earn billions of dollars annually from this illicit trade—and who would rapidly lose their competitive advantage if marijuana were a legal commodity."

Like opium and willow tree bark, the active ingredient in marijuana beneficial in fighting pain grows in nature—but in this case as a "weed." Labeled by the United Nations as the "most widely used illicit substance in the world," marijuana creates a powerful psychoactive chemical compound commonly known as THC—but which goes by the scientific name of Tetrahydrocannabinol.

Biologists believe that marijuana, known to some researchers as "cannabis," naturally developed THC as a defensive mechanism, perhaps to fight off herbivores or organisms that eat plants. According to a 2009 article in "Archives of General Psychiatry," a whopping 400 different chemical compounds are in cannabis. In fact, a 2006 "New York Free Press" article, "Lost Civilizations of the Stone Age," said some people began using marijuana as far back as 3,000 years before Christ.

Anthropologists have found evidence of cannabis use thousands of years ago in such diverse places as China, Bulgaria, Greece and early Iran. Whether these early cultures used marijuana to kill or block pain remains a matter of dispute. Although marijuana is much less powerful than opium and opiate-based drugs, various countries began to criminalize cannabis through the early 1900s including New Zealand, the United Kingdom, Jamaica and South Africa. In 1906, authorities in Washington, D.C., imposed restrictions on cannabis, and the U.S. Congress passed the "Marihuana Tax Act," placing a tax on the sale of cannabis, while prohibiting the production of marijuana and its byproduct, hemp.

Cannabis Offers Numerous Well-Documented Benefits

Although the use of marijuana for medicinal purposes remains controversial, numerous studies cite its effectiveness as an analgesic or pain reliever, according to various medical studies. Researchers also insist that their studies indicate the effectiveness of cannabis in treating glaucoma, and AIDS—while also stimulating hunger in cancer patients as they undergo chemotherapy.

Despite such findings, the U.S. Food and Drug Administration, commonly known as the FDA, has not authorized the use of marijuana for medical purposes. Meantime, a federal law enforcement agency, the Drug Enforcement Administration or DEA pursues those who distribute or produce marijuana with the same ferocity as "heavy" drugs like heroin and cocaine.

Criminalizing "possession of a drug should not be more damaging to an individual than the use of the drug itself, and where they are they should be charged," said Jimmy Carter, 39th president of the United States from 1977 to 1981. Despite such political convictions, the severity and potential harmfulness remains a matter of dispute involving specific drug types—especially marijuana.

Cannabis can be administered in a variety of methods, most often smoking, inhaling or eating when baked into common foods such as brownies. Meantime, while the use of marijuana for medical purposes remains a highly disputed hot political topic, such activities are deemed legally permissible in only a limited number of countries and states.

Fighting Pain with Marijuana is a Moral Choice

The question of whether to use marijuana in medicine remains a hot moral issue as people argue sharply diverse opinions. Yet society needs to realize that literally all highly powerful pain killing medications remain extremely powerful and potentially dangerous, not just cannabis.

By recent accounts, the use of marijuana via prescription for legitimate medical purposes is allowed in varying degrees in at least 16 states including California, by far the most populous of them. And, the Golden State is among seven that authorize dispensaries for medically prescribed cannabis; the others are Michigan, Montana, Rhode Island, Maine, New Mexico and Colorado.

Complicating matters, however, from the view of federal officials marijuana remains an illegal drug. And the federal Food and Drug Administration, commonly called the "FDA," has issued a controversial advisory stating that while marijuana is subject to abuse, there is "no currently accepted medical use (of marijuana) in treatment in the United States." According to some published reports, the only instance where the FDA authorizes the medical use of cannabis is in oral form as dronabinol or nabilone. These are sometimes used only after other standard treatments fail to work in alleviating adverse symptoms such as nausea and vomiting associated with chemotherapy.

Paradoxically, selling marijuana still remains illegal under federal law, even in the wake of a 2009 U.S. Justice Department memo to all state attorneys general. The document provided seven criteria that prosecutors can use when determining to pursue criminal action in specific medical marijuana cases. At the same time, though, federal officials recommended against prosecuting patients who have followed state laws in receiving and using such prescriptions.

One of the most common criticisms stemmed from concerns that the process of smoking cannabis would threaten the patients' health. Advocates of such treatments insist that doctors have managed to efficiently and legally sidestep such concerns thanks to much safer consumption methods such as inhaling marijuana aroma processed through a vaporizer, or when eating THC-laden food.

Willie Nelson, a popular American musician and entertainer, has been quoted as saying that "I think people need to be educated to the fact that marijuana is not a drug. Marijuana is an herb and a flower. God put it here. If he put it here and he wants it to grow, what gives the government the right to say that God is wrong?"

On the so-called flip side of this proverbial coin, though, some law enforcement officials still insist that marijuana even for medical use is a "doorway drug," opening up the possibility that an individual will become addicted to much more harmful substances.

Study the Facts Before Deciding Whether to Use Medical Marijuana

From my view, many people fake illnesses or seek phony cannabis prescriptions just so they can abuse marijuana as a recreational drug. Overall, this stems from the same potentially harmful process that lots of consumers use to obtain extremely harmful and dangerously addictive pain-killing drugs produced by pharmaceutical companies and dispersed by local pharmacies.

Ultimately, the decision on whether to legally use marijuana for medical reasons should not be taken lightly by patients or physicians. Doctors have a moral and professional responsibility to only prescribe drugs for legitimate and useful reasons as medical treatments.

With this in mind, I recommend that patients pursuing or considering the possibility of marijuana prescriptions to take the following precautions at the very least:

- Prognosis: Is your current medical condition or pain truly significant, to the point where you would want to even consider using such a substance?

- Alternatives: Before pursuing or even considering such a prescription, patients should study the possibility of other more traditional medications, herbs or lifestyles. An oral prescription form of THC is available for patients suffering from nausea, vomiting and anorexia.

- Reputation: Study the background, education and overall reputation of the physician who might prescribe marijuana for you. Does he or she have a good reputation for issuing such treatments only in specific, essential instances?

- Cost: Some patients, especially those with low incomes, also might feel a need to research potential costs for marijuana prescriptions. Be sure to check whether your insurance company covers the cost of such drugs. And, if not, you should ponder whether the potential benefit would be worth the expense.

- Abuse: As a physician, I always recommend that patients strive to avoid abusing drugs of any kind ranging from alcohol to highly illegal narcotics. Anyone striving to obtain such a prescription merely in order to abuse marijuana should seek to get professional help, either by first inquiring with a physician or visiting organizations such as Narcotics Anonymous.

While approaching this possibility from a serious and thoughtful perspective, some patients also might want to keep in mind that serious research has indicated the medical use of marijuana generates definite benefits—at least in some specific instances.

A 2009 article in the "Journal of Clinical Investigation" said that in some studies marijuana use was effective in killing harmful brain cancer cells while leaving healthy cells intact within the organ. Another 2009 article on the PhysOrg.com Web site cited a study concluding that stressed rats injected with the THC byproduct of cannabis became less dependant on opiates. And according to media reports at least one other study indicated the apparent effectiveness of marijuana in lessening the muscular spasms and swelling sometimes suffered by people with multiple sclerosis.

When referring to marijuana, the late Nobel Prize-winning economist and statistician of the 20th Century, Milton Friedman, said, "When a private enterprise fails, it is closed down; when a government enterprise fails, it is expanded. Isn't that exactly what is happening with drugs?"

Chapter 30

Scientists Developed a Vast Array of Analgesics

B acked by research and scientific developments through thousands of years and many wars, through the 20th Century physicians helped create and embraced a vast array of pain-killing pharmaceuticals called "analgesics." For the most part these are comprised of opium-based products such as morphine, and also salicylate or salicylic acid-based products derived from willow tree bark such as aspirin.

In a majority of cases, physicians choose specific analgesics depending on the diagnosed severity of pain stemming from specific types of wounds or illness. Yet, analgesics are not effective for all types of pain, such as certain instances of neuropathic pain that occur as a result of certain types of lesions, specific disorders within the peripheral nervous system such as in the spinal cord or brain, or in specific types of cancers. Other potential factors include complications following chemotherapy, diabetic neuropathies, and post-herpetic neuropathy.

Thus, although the most frequently used pain-killing category, medications within the general spectrum of analgesics are not designed to cover all types of physical pain. In addition, it is also important for patients to remember that the analgesics category should not be confused with anesthetics—pharmaceuticals administered only by medical professionals to eliminate sensations during major surgeries or for much less serious medical procedures such as dentistry, the removal of toenails by podiatrists or minor surgical procedures.

Patients who want to know the basics of the analgesic category of choices often find it easy to understand the primary classes or subsets within this realm. They are:

- Paracetamol: Also known as NSAIDs, these are non-steroidal and anti-inflammatory drugs like aspirin. As an overall category, paracetamol generates fewer side-effects than much more powerful analgesics, while also usually lacking the propensity for dangerous addictions. Despite extensive advances in overall science, researchers still fail to understand how this substance works in all instances. Numerous studies indicate these substances work centrally within the brain rather than on nerve endings. Despite its ranking as relatively safe compared to much more powerful analgesics, overuse of paracetamol can damage the upper gastrointestinal tract, the liver, or generate a variety of physical problems such as hearing loss, kidney damage and allergic reactions. In addition, especially among children, some people suffer from Reye's Syndrome fever, a severe allergy to aspirin that can cause potentially fatal brain and liver disease.

- COX-2 Inhibitors: Developed largely by pharmaceutical companies, these are generally derived from the same substances used to create aspirin, created largely in an effort to block specific types of enzymes in order to develop less gastrointestinal hemorrhaging. This compares to aspirin, which sometimes causes stomach ulcerations or digestive tract problems, especially when ingested regularly on an empty stomach. Despite the advantages of COX-2 inhibitors, this substance also poses an array of potential physical setbacks, according to various published reports. These include the possibility of cardiac problems or brain-area difficulties. COX-2 inhibitors have also been used in the treatment of colorectal cancers as adjuvant therapies.

- Opiates: Also including morphine and various other drugs, this is among the most powerful but potentially addictive range within analgesics. Despite the extremely powerful pain-killing attributes within the opiate and morphinomimetics range, this class can result in many potentially unpleasant side effects. Besides the risk of itching and constipation, these drugs also pose the potential problems of vomiting and nausea. Thus, many physicians also prescribe additional medications such as laxatives when treating patients with this type of analgesic. Some of the most common drugs within the opiate and morphine-based category are:

  - Codeine: Extracted from opium poppies, this is generally considered within the weak or mid-range level of the opiate class. The specific ingredients of codeine are made from only a small portion of the numerous active ingredients from the poppies. According to at least some published accounts, codeine has just 8 percent to 12 percent of the overall pain-fighting strength of morphine. Usually taken orally as a pill, codeine is often considered less addictive than morphine and is most often prescribed for mild or moderate pain. Codeine is sometimes sold under brand names such as Vicodin™ when intermixed with lower-dose acetominaphen. The potential adverse effects of codeine can include everything from euphoria, depression and constipation to nausea, drowsiness, itching, rashes, and other complications.

- Oxycodone: Also primarily comprised from a specific active ingredient produced by opium poppies, this is categorized as a "semi-synthetic" because the drug is produced when compounding isolated substances from within natural sources. Sometimes sold under the time-released brand name OxyContin® produced by Purdue Pharma—the rights remaining under dispute—this also is available in generic form. Historians of drug research say scientists in Germany discovered or isolated oxycodone in 1916, and scientists subsequently achieved at least some of their objective of generating this as a less-addictive alternative to heroin. Under the brand name OxyContin®, use increased sharply from the mid-1990s through the first decade of the 21st Century, and according to news reports the manufacturer changed the formula in 2010 in attempts to decrease misuse of this drug. In recent years, the news media has reported various marketing and branding issues involving OxyContin®. Meantime, at least seven other brand names with varying related compounds have been marketed and distributed. Besides euphoria and memory loss, the various potential side effects of oxycodone can include everything from nausea and dizziness to headaches, anxiety and more intense side effects of codeine.

- Hydrocodone: Also a semi-synthetic and derived from opium, as a specific ingredient found within the poppies, this pain killer is often taken in the form of a tablet or as a syrup to depress coughs. Some scientists debate the effectiveness of hydrocodone, particularly when taken without other analgesics. Nonetheless, at least judging by some published accounts, hydrocodone might be at least two times more effective than standard codeine. First approved by the FDA in 1943 for U.S. sales, initially under the brand name Hycocan™, hydrocodone eventually got manufactured, distributed and sold under at least 20 brand names. Although deemed stronger than codeine but with only one tenth of morphine's strength, this drug poses the potential of harmful addiction. As a result, physicians sometimes prescribe this only under strict supervision with drugs designed to counteract some potentially harmful effects, or with other analgesics. Used for mild to moderate pain, hydrocodone can generate severe negative reactions when mixed with certain other drugs like alcohol, barbiturates or cocaine. Its side effects include those of codeine.

- Dihydromorphine: Physicians describe this as very similar to morphine, sometimes even stronger than that drug—acting faster and lasting longer. Also an opiate, this semi-synthetic was discovered in 1900, at least a generation before some of its less powerful counterparts. Partly as a result of this drug's extreme strength, the U.S. government considers dihydromorphine as an extremely dangerous "Schedule 1" narcotic. Its specific strength when compared to morphine, whether less or more effective, remains in dispute among researchers. It is marketed under the name Dilaudid™.

- Pethidine: Commonly called "Demerol," but also referred to by a wide variety of other names, this opiate analgesic is sometimes termed as a "meperidine." Heralded as fast-acting and first introduced in 1932, this was considered as the opiate that many physicians preferred when prescribing opium-based medications during much of the 20th Century. But perhaps because some physicians consider pethidine as no more effective than morphine, this drug decreased in popularity while being severely restricted in some countries such as Australia. Considered highly addictive, its possible severe potential side effects include tremors, seizures, and "dysphoria," a term for uncontrollably unpleasant moods. This analgesic is seldom used in oncology.

- Flupirtine: While not an opiate, unrelated to willow tree barks, and not steroid-based, this drug first introduced by Asta Medica in Europe in 1984 for pain treatment has never been introduced in the United States. In 2008, the Adeona pharmacy acquired an option to license the pending and issued patents for Flupirtine, while scientists research its possible effectiveness as a treatment for Alzheimer's Disease, multiple sclerosis, and fibromyalgia, a medical disorder that results in muscular and connective tissue pain.

Other specific agents: In addition to the aspirin-like and opiate-based drugs in the analgesic category, a variety of other substances are sometimes either used or considered, according to at least some reports. These might include specific types of anti-depressants or tricyclic antidepressants. In most instances, as the description implies, this is used to relieve the symptoms of depression. Meantime, certain anti-depressants are sometimes also prescribed for the treatment of chronic pain. Nefopam™, first developed as an opiate alternative in the early 1970s, is widely used but mostly in Europe. Much stronger at fighting pain than aspirin, Nefopam™ sometimes causes sweating, dizziness and nausea, while deemed half as potent as oxycodone and morphine.

Chapter 31

Physicians Use the Ladder of Pain

Following a tradition or system first embraced by oncologists, many physicians use what the general public sometimes calls the "pain ladder." For the most part this process usually entails starting at the bottom of the proverbial ladder, initially prescribing low-dose or less addictive drugs with minimal side effects such as aspirin or the equivalent of common over-the-counter drugs.

When and if a particular phase or step such as the lower-rung aspirin level fails to mask or eliminate pain, the physician might consider prescribing a stronger analgesic. At the top rung, the least-used option involves full-fledged opiate-class pharmaceuticals.

The middle-rungs often involve weak or increasingly strong opiates, plus potential combinations of other drugs such as aspirin or over-the-counter products.

The ultimate objective is to prescribe super-strong and highly addictive opiates only when necessary. And conversely, as pain eventually lessens, an illness subsides or a wound heals, physicians can step down this proverbial pain ladder. This way doctors steadily begin administering the less potent medications.

"Champions keep playing until they get it right," said Billy Jean King, a former professional tennis star, a Wimbledon champion who in 1972 became the first female named athlete of the year by "Sports Illustrated."

Doctors Administer a Combination of Analgesics

Physicians and pharmaceutical companies often administer a combination of analgesics, depending on the specific severity of pain or the illness involved. For instance, remedies might include over-the-counter analgesics along with antihistamines to fight flu symptoms such as fever, muscle pains, a runny nose and watery eyes.

But many physicians warn any efforts to mix drugs should be done with extreme caution. According to a 2010 article in the "Australian Prescriber," combining analgesics can sometimes generate confusion and result in accidental overdoses when using multiple drugs, some not necessary or not intended for the patient's specific symptoms.

In addition, rather than orally or via injection, some analgesics such as ibuprofen, capsaicin and diclofenac are administered as gels— rubbed onto the body's surface at the site of painful muscles or joints. Meantime, physicians sometimes inject steroids or the anesthetic Lidocaine™ into painful joints to generate long-term pain relief.

Adding to their many options, some doctors seeking to relieve or mask pain also administer anticholinergic agents, any substance that blocks neurotransmitters within the body's central nervous system. These range from Orphenadrin in treating painful muscle spasms to Cyclobenzaprine, a muscle relaxant medication.

The many so-called atypical or adjuvant analgesics add diversity and complexity to the diverse options available to physicians. Some of these treatments are intended to modify the effects of specific medications, while never giving any of their own direct effects.

Physicians and Patients Use a Popular Reference Book

The widely popular and highly respected "Physicians Desk Reference" serves as a bible or dictionary on a vast range of pain killers and medications for various illnesses. Commonly called "The PDR," this regularly updated book features a description of all primary, basic or advanced pain killers and other pharmaceutical products made by the major drug companies.

Available in bookstores, libraries and via Web connections to subscribers, the PDR serves as a valuable reference source for physicians, a wide range of medical professionals and by consumers curious about drugs they currently use or might get. Most descriptions feature images of the actual pills or products.

Certainly, this book for basic knowledge can help satisfy the curiosity of patients interested in inquiring about the many countless specific pain medications. However, you should remember that if and when using this publication, keep in mind that the most powerful pain medications used in the mainstream allopathic medical industry can only be issued by a licensed physicians. As always, I can't seem to stress enough that patients should never attempt to diagnose their own illnesses.

Despite what experts cite as the many advantages of the PDR, some patients remain cognizant that the publication lacks integral information on many of the basic natural substances often prescribed by homeopaths. The vast majority of the natural products that homeopaths recommend are not amassed, distributed or sold by the world's largest pharmaceutical companies.

Other critics of the PDR also complain that some listings on specific drugs are incomplete, or that data on numerous individual pharmaceuticals is sometimes listed before researchers have finished integral studies on new or developing medications. Adding heat to the issue, some observers contend that pharmaceutical companies often supply the PDR's producers with information that sometimes lacks details on potential negative side effects. In every yearly edition the PDR allows for "off-label" use of every drug listed.

From my view, for patients the PDR is best suited as a basic reference guide, in essence a dictionary for determining basic details on what they're either already taking or what a physician prescribes or recommends for them. As a patient, you should always feel free to ask your doctor or pharmacy professionals for the specifics on any drug you're taking such as recommended precautions such as whether to avoid meals or driving.

"The important thing is not to stop questioning," said Albert Einstein, the 20th Century genius. "Curiosity has its own reason for existing."

Chapter 32

Anesthesia Produces Essential Pain-Killing for Surgeries

Patients who undergo anything from a basic outpatient procedure such as dental work to extensive surgery usually needs what doctors call an anesthetic, sometimes spelled "anaesthetic." For the most part these drugs create what doctors call the "reversible loss of sensation."

Except for extreme or rare instances, anesthetic pharmaceuticals are not used to deaden or block pain during non-surgical periods. For less extensive procedures, licensed professionals such as dentists working on teeth or podiatrists extracting toenails administer lower-dose anesthetics during outpatient procedures performed in their clinics.

The situation is much more extensive and poses even greater potential dangers for complex surgeries such as operations performed in hospitals. For many of the most complex procedures, surgeons often work with the assistance of specialized anesthesiologists. Such licensed and highly educated professionals administer specific types of powerful anesthetics.

When administered correctly, powerful anesthetics used in surgeries put the patient in a sleep-like state for a limited period. Extremely serious complications and even death can occur if such drugs are administered incorrectly, or when such patients fail to receive continuous monitoring by a certified anesthesiologist. Authorities say the abuse of high-powered anesthetics is extremely rare, largely due to the extreme danger involved.

Perhaps the most famous case of such apparent abuse involved the late entertainment superstar Michael Jackson, at least according to criminal prosecutors. Jackson died at age 50 in June 2009 in what the Los Angeles Coroner's Office listed as a homicide involving a powerful anesthetic. Jackson's personal physician, Conrad Murray, pleaded not guilty to criminal manslaughter charges. News stories quoted Jackson's acquaintances as saying the restless star abused analgesics in order to get much-needed sleep.

The Jackson case should serve as an urgent example to all sufferers of intense pain that they should never consider or try any form of anesthetic in an attempt to administer at-home relief for sleep problems. Even physicians say the in-home use of such powerful anesthetics is ill-advised, extremely dangerous and unnecessary, even when administered by a doctor. For patients suffering from sleep problems, physicians have a wide range of other much more sensible treatments or lifestyle changes.

Anesthetics Fall within Specified Classifications

Pharmacists and medical professionals list anesthetics within two primary classifications. The first, "general anesthetics," puts patients in a temporary unconsciousness during significant medical procedures such as surgery. The "local anesthetics" category generates a temporary loss of sensation in a specific part of the body while patients remain awake.

In addition to general and local anesthetics, the anesthesia branch of medicine features two additional classifications that are not often in the public mindset. The first of these is "regional anesthetics" where an entire section of the body such as a limb is treated to induce a loss of sensation. Doctors sometimes use a catheter to continuously inject anesthetic drugs into a specific area of the body, such as epidural procedures performed upon the onset of childbirth's final stage, or for a caesarian section.

Medical experts consider the application of regional anesthetics as potentially more dangerous than local anesthetics that are done in extremely limited bodily areas such as the fingers, toes or teeth. Possible complications from regional procedures include seizures, cardiac arrest or spinal shock where many physical sensations are blocked for extended periods.

Due to these possible dangers, in case of a medical emergency, physicians performing regional procedures such as localized operations on limbs are sometimes prepared to immediately revert to general anesthesia impacting the entire body.

As a result of these dangers, many regional anesthetic procedures like extensive facelift operations are done in extremely safe conditions. Although such surgeries are often performed within a doctor's office, such facilities frequently provide highly trained personnel capable of administering general anesthetics.

For minor procedures that need local anesthetics, medical professionals have a choice from at least ten substances that block the ability of nerves to transmit the sensation of pain. Many doctors prefer to avoid three of these options because they are considered unstable while also often resulting in allergic reactions—cocaine, procaine and amethocaine. This leaves the remaining options, each ending in the phrase "caine," indicating that the effective substances render cellular communications or interactions via the nervous system, rendering those sections of the body ineffective for limited periods.

In both general anesthetics and local anesthetics the term "anesthesia" is used to describe what occurs when the doctor intentionally induces either of three reversible states or conditions:

- Amnesia: A temporary loss of memory.

- Analgesia: The temporary elimination of responsiveness from sensations including pain, while also decreasing skeletal muscle reflexes and responses to stress.

- Multi-effects: A variety of some, or all, of the above-listed temporary outcomes.

Before any scheduled medical procedures requiring local or general anesthetics, patients should feel free to ask questions about how the surgery is performed.

Dissociative Anesthetics Impact the Mental Process

Besides local, general and regional anesthetics, doctors also sometimes use "dissociative anesthetics" in a specified effort to block or curtail the transmission of pain signals from the conscious mind to various areas of the brain.

Many of these narcotics, some of them addictive, produce hallucinogenic effects. The related possible side effects range from sensory depravation to trances or "dream-like states," and even a sense of dissociation—when the mind feels distanced from the physical realm. The level, duration and occurrence of these specific conditions are often unpredictable and challenging for almost any physician to foresee.

These behaviors or reactions sometimes strike patients and even seasoned medical professionals who care for them as rather unsettling. Some patients, even those striving to fight off pain, end up behaving in unanticipated ways far different from their usual lifestyle patterns.

"Behavior is a mirror in which everyone displays his own image," said Johann Wolfgang von Goethe, a 19th Century German polymath and writer, heralded as an extreme genius and highly adept at many endeavors including drama, literature and science.

Besides intentionally via the use of narcotics or anesthetics, the occurrence of dissociative mental reactions sometimes erupts as a result of trauma or mental abuse. Such causes increase the complexity of challenging symptoms among patients recovering from such trauma as gunshot wounds or sexual attacks.

Most doctors avoid prescribing psychoactive drugs in any attempt to alleviate or block physical pain, at least from my perspective as a medical professional. The many substances that generate dissociative properties can range from LSD and alcohol to PCP and atropine—all within the category of psychoactive drugs. Despite the many potential drawbacks, such substances sometimes result in blocking or warding off extreme physical or emotional pain.

Many Types of Plants Generate Primary Anesthetic Products

Many of the world's largest pharmaceutical companies use derivatives from plants around the world to generate anesthetic drugs accepted and used by mainstream physicians. Although known today primarily as a highly addictive and extremely dangerous narcotic, in the mid-1800s cocaine was sometimes used as an anesthetic.

After inhaled or inhalational anesthetics such as diethyl ether were first introduced in 1846—initially for dentistry—and chloroform, many of the anesthetic drugs used most frequently today for a wide variety of medical procedures were gradually approved by the medical industry during the following 150 years.

The emergence of these new life-saving technologies gradually resulted in the increasingly accepted and even the required medical specialty of anesthesiologists. These highly trained medical professionals devote their careers to providing and implementing anesthetics in the safest conditions possible. According to a 2010 report by the American Society of Anesthesiologists, of the more than 40 million annual medical procedures requiring anesthetics, such professionals provided or administered anesthesia in 90 percent of the cases.

In the United States, in order to become fully certified, anesthesiologists must undergo at least four years of residency or post-graduate medical training in their specialty—starting after they graduate from medical school. Thus, like general physicians and highly specialized practices such as oncology, these professionals must excel through a minimum combined 12 years of college and post-graduate education after high school.

In addition, in the United States some hospitals or medical facilities also employ "certified registered nurse anesthetists" or CRNAs. Many of these nurses work for anesthesiologists, hospitals, surgeons, podiatrists, dentists, obstetricians and other medical professionals who regularly render anesthetics.

Anesthesiologists have emerged as so integral to the medical and recovery process that such specialists also are recruited to work in non-surgical settings. Their work often proves essential before, during and after operations. Such doctors strive to ensure that patients maintain a stable and constant physical condition, everything from variations in bodily temperatures to the overall functioning of organs to ensure blood sugar levels and the production of urine remains healthy.

The Highly Specialized Medicine of Anesthetics Remains Vital

Increasingly during the 20th Century and particularly during the past several decades, anesthetics has become so specialized and essential to the success of overall medical care that many facilities also employ "anesthesia technicians." In much the way that scrub technicians assist surgeons, an anesthesia technician performs essential duties for anesthesiologists.

As seen in popular TV shows and in the movies, high-level anesthetic equipment features extensive, complex and often essential machines ranging from vaporizers to pressure gauges and ventilators. A malfunction of any or all of these devices could result in a medical emergency, such as the malfunction of a vital machine part or the unintentional transmission of harmful bacteria to the patient—risking serious or even fatal infections.

Adding to the complexity, throughout extensive medical procedures and surgeries anesthesiologists are responsible for continually monitoring a patient's vital signs. All essential bodily functions are tracked, from the heart rate to blood pressure, EKG and EEG monitoring, oxygen levels, and the intake or output of gasses.

As if these many urgent tasks weren't already enough in the overall process of blocking pain, especially during critical surgeries the vast team of doctors and nurses depends on anesthesiologists to monitor pressures within blood vessels. When any of these vital signs malfunctions, these doctors work with the entire medical crew to re-stabilize the patient. Seasoned and well-trained professionals take these responsibilities in stride, responding to specific types of emergencies in pre-defined, step-by-step manners—following an exact protocol.

"Out of intense complexities intense simplicities emerge," said Sir Winston Churchill, the 20th Century British prime minister.

Particularly in what many physicians call today's "suit-happy society," where some patients file frivolous law suits against hospitals and doctors, anesthesiologists also get saddled with the additional responsibility of keeping intricate, highly detailed and minute-to-minute records of what transpired during each major surgical procedure.

The need to keep lawyers at bay has resulted in this vital information-gathering process, playing a significant role in shooting up overall medical costs. Even for standard surgeries the necessary data includes full lists of administered drugs, when and how much they were given, the intake and output of fluids, specific amounts of blood loss, and even all of the various vital sign readings recorded throughout the operation.

Despite the additional work and expense required, this massive data often serves an essential and vital purpose in advancing the knowledge of medical experts. For instance, doctors can use data on specific phase-by-phase improvements in many patients to determine the best ways to fight pain and to devise the most effective treatments.

Some Patients Report They Remain Alert and Aware of Pain During Surgery

Shockingly, at least judging by numerous stories in recent years in the mainstream news media, some patients who underwent surgery claimed they remained fully alert and feeling intense pain during their operations. Some observers have termed this condition as "anesthesia awareness" or "unintended intra-operative awareness."

In at least some cases, patients claim that medical professionals failed to give them enough anesthetic to render them fully unconscious during surgery. Could many of these patients be confused, wrongly believing that what they sensed while regaining consciousness in the recovery room had actually occurred during their surgeries?

Beginning early in this century, some published reports have estimated that from 0.01% to 0.02% or about one or two out of every 10,000 people who undergo surgery claim to have remained in a state of awareness during the procedure.

Once again, here, I feel a need to state my professional opinion. Reports of such instances need much more study before physicians can make any conclusive statements on the issue. Before any of my patients undergoes surgery, if they might happen to inquire, I would tell them that any instance of anesthesia awareness remains extremely unlikely. For more than a century, anesthesiologists have developed pre-specified systems of determining the amount of drugs needed to render a person fully unconscious—largely dependant on the person's body weight and overall physical structure.

Also on the positive side, only about one third to nearly one half of those who claim to remain aware during surgery reported that they felt any pain, at least judging by some published reports. Understandably, nearly all of those who claimed to have felt pain—a full 94 percent of them—claimed that they suffered from anxiety or panic, in some instances experiencing difficulty breathing.

Some Patients Are Intentionally Kept Awake During Surgery

Patients commonly remain awake during local anesthesia for minor in-office, outpatient surgeries. A much less common practice occurs when physicians intentionally keep the patient awake during some major operations.

During some brain operations, for instance, surgeons strive to keep patients fully cognizant during the procedures in order to signal to doctors what they feel—if anything—when a specific part of the body gets touched. These procedures also can serve as an essential way for the patient to communicate, or to specify whether various regions of the body are functioning as planned.

Much of the credit for these advancements should go to the overall profession of anesthesiology, as physicians continually strive for vital advancements in pain-relieving medicines and technologies.

Chapter 33

Steroids Also Play a Huge Role

M ost of the mainstream publicity that involves steroids erupts from the illegal, ill-advised or dangerous use of such substances by athletes. However, many people throughout the general public fail to realize steroids also can play a vital role in legitimate medicine, particularly in eradicating painful conditions.

Understandably, steroids get a much-deserved bad rap because many of these substances are known carcinogens. However, when used in prescribed medical conditions under a doctor's supervision, steroids can alleviate or lessen painful conditions such as certain lung problems, muscular diseases or arthritis conditions.

Steroids are either synthetically created by pharmaceutical companies, or they are derived from plants. Within the human body, steroids occur naturally. Part of the problem that steroids pose stems from the fact that when used as drugs they're administered in highly concentrated amounts, often far more than the body normally uses.

The human body naturally generates many types of hormones, ranging from sex hormones that regulate everything from the libido to reproductive tendencies.

Some hormones also possess anti-inflammatory characteristics, often ideal for eliminating painful symptoms. Nonetheless, steroids also can emerge as highly destructive within the bodies of athletes striving to artificially build or retain muscle mass.

Anabolic Steroids and Others Play a Critical Role

Besides features affecting sexual functions and cholesterol levels, within the class of vertebrate steroids that impact creatures with backbones there are two integral subsets involving pain:

- Anabolic steroids: These impact the muscles, sex organs, and bones, hinging on androgen receptors by using natural or synthetic substances.

- Corticosteroids: These impact everything from stress levels to immune system responses, levels of inflammation and behavior, including "fight or flight" responses.

Due to the extreme power and potential dangers of these substances, the possession and use of many specific types of anabolic steroids and corticosteroids in drug form is illegal unless under the prescription of a licensed physician. A patient seeking relief of pain should never under any circumstances attempt to obtain and use such substances outside of a doctor's care. Besides cancer, the potential life-threatening or debilitating long-term consequences of corticosteroids include cataracts, insulin resistant diabetes mellitus, permanent eye damage from glaucoma, depression, anxiety, muscle weakness, immune suppression, central obesity and "striae," commonly known as "stretch marks."

Within the corticosteroid class, synthetic glucocorticoids are often used in legitimate medicine to relieve debilitating conditions that cause joint pain and inflammation—primarily involving arthritis, dermatitis, asthma, cancers, and many other ailments. Many of these medical advances clicked into gear in the mid-1900s, particularly when three physicians won the Nobel Prize in physiology and medicine. Tadeusz Reichstein, Edward Calvin Kendall and Philip Showalter Hench earned much-deserved recognition for their groundbreaking work that enabled scientists to isolate cortisone.

Cortisone Enabled Physicians to Hit a Grand Slam Against Pain

Thanks largely to the isolation of cortisone made possible in part by the significant contributions of Kendall, a researcher at the Mayo Clinic, Merck & Company began producing cortisone in the 1950s. As the end-product of an extensive, complex biological process that involves the adrenal glands, the body produces "cortisol," a natural response to stress that increasing blood sugar levels. Meantime, while suppressing the immune system, cortisol also assists in various metabolism functions that involve carbohydrates, fats and proteins.

Scientists list cortisone as an inactive metabolite of cortisol. When produced naturally within the body, cortisone serves as nature's way of reacting to stress. This is the same process that erupts during an extreme emergency, such as when the body prepares for a "flight or fight" mode, sometimes giving people extreme and unexpected strength in running away from their adversaries or even in order to battle their opponents.

Doctors sometimes employ this technique, generating short-term pain relief by injecting cortisone directly into an affected or swollen joint or tendon such as the knee, shoulder and elbow. Patients who had suffered extreme, excruciating pain in those areas often proclaim that cortisone is a "miracle" immediately after receiving such treatments.

"My knee had hurt so bad that I once couldn't walk or move," said Patricia, a patient who recently received cortisone for her persistent condition. "Right after the shot, everything was better right away and the pain subsided."

Like many other patients, Patricia also was advised to take proactive lifestyle changes in order to treat her underlying condition. Thereafter, at least five days a week she exercised in the swimming pool of an exercise facility, and the pain never returned for several years. But her knee pain slowly began to re-emerge after a necessary operation to remove an ingrown toenail; the recovery period from that procedure prevented her from engaging in her favorite exercise routine for more than one month.

Understandably, Patricia resumed her exercise regimen as soon as possible, once again enabling her knee pain to subside. Her story serves as just one example that short-term pain killing remedies such as cortisone should not be considered as the only solution to eradicating pain. Ultimately, when working under the advice of their patients, many patients suffering from chronic pain need to engage in consistent physical therapy or vital and consistent exercise routines.

Meantime, cortisone should never be considered as the one-and-only drug for treating such pains. Like all other potentially powerful medications or substances, this steroid derivative poses numerous negative side effects due to its impact on the immune system. Potential myocardial arrests and excessive fluid in the abdomen are among dangers.

James W. Forsythe, M.D., H.M.D.

Anabolic Steroids Remain
Highly Controversial

Another subset within this class, anabolic steroids, remains highly controversial due to the extreme dangers involved, coupled with use by professional athletes.

While mirroring the effects of male sex hormones such as testosterone, anabolic steroids generate masculine qualities like excessive hair, deepened voices and expansive muscles.

Since scientists first identified, isolated and began creating synthetic versions of anabolic steroids in the 1930s, the controversy has stirred and never seems to subside. Just some of the many potential dangerous side effects when used long-term include damage to the heart's left ventricle and severe or life-threatening liver damage.

As mentioned in several of my other best-selling books, including one endorsed by superstar media personality Suzanne Somers, some of the world's most popular sports heroes have abused anabolic steroids to get a competitive edge. Even before researchers isolated these substances, called "gonadal steroids," in the 1800s physicians began studying extracts from the testicles. In the late 1930s, bodybuilders and weightlifters were among the first athletes to begin abusing anabolic steroids.

Covertly, many athletes liked the way these steroids generated proteins to increase muscle mass, while also blocking the negative impacts of stress on muscles. When used under careful and authorized medical supervision, anabolic steroids can help improve or relieve the painful side effects of such ailments as osteoporosis and traumas caused by surgeries or extensive periods of remaining motionless.

Meantime, doctors and their patients need to remain aware of the potential adverse psychiatric effects, which can include mood disorders and substance abuse. Highly aggressive behaviors sometimes occur, often called "roid rage" that has been known to result in manic characteristics, physically abusive behavior, and even suicide.

Despite these many undeniable problems, physicians have used anabolic steroids for lots of specific pain-related treatments with varying degrees of success. Besides treating various forms of anemias, other conditions include arthritis, kidney failure, leukemia, and breast cancer; these substances can also stimulate growth and appetite.

Even in the midst of such potential benefits, virtually every significant professional sports organization bans the use of anabolic steroids, including Major League Baseball, the National Football League and the National Basketball Association.

Chapter 34

Neurology Remains Integral in the Detection and Relief of Pain

A vital medical specialty commonly called neurology often performs an integral role in the detection, diagnosis and potential elimination of pain. This branch of medicine is integral to practicing neurologists who focus on any disorder within the body's entire nervous structures—the autonomic, central and peripheral nervous systems.

Since the nervous system plays an essential role in communicating the signals of pain from various areas of the body to the brain, neurologists often are sought after as a first-line of analysis, diagnosis and detection as they devise and implement treatments. And, within the realm, neurosurgeons often perform necessary surgical procedures.

The role of neurologists in pain-related specialties within standard medicine handle everything from performing or managing research for pharmaceutical companies to conducting clinical trials of current or proposed painkillers. All these many tasks involve "neuroscience," the science and study of the body's nervous system.

Besides pain-related medical conditions such as gunshot wounds or even the ravages of advanced arthritis, these physicians often identify and treat many types of neurological disorders. These range from paralysis to muscle weaknesses, to seizures and other adverse characteristics that often result in extreme pain. Many of these problems stem from chemical or electrical abnormalities, some inherited. According to various published reports, the World Health Organization has estimated that at least 1 billion people, or nearly one out of every seven people has at least one type of neurological disorder.

Thus, people suffering from strange or seemingly unexplainable pains often get their first definitive "answers" about their conditions after finally seeing a neurologist. Many problems stem from abnormalities within the brain, spinal cord or nervous systems.

Thankfully, once a neurologist has located and specified a specific nerve-related cause to a painful disorder, he or she can then strive to issue the best-possible treatments. Possible adverse conditions or symptoms include migraine headaches, sleep disorders and certain types of back pain. Some neurologists choose to specialize in any of a vast range of disorders, such as dementia, epilepsy and multiple sclerosis.

Many Neurologists Try to Dismiss the Legitimacy of Homeopathic Medicine

While locked into the practice of so-called mainstream traditional medicine, most neurologists scoff at or strive to trivialize today's practitioners of homeopathic medicine. Overall, homeopathy entails the use of natural substances such as plant extracts or herbs for the treatment of physical ailments. Taking a sharply different course, standard-practice neurologists usually prescribe only synthetic or mass-produced drugs that are made and distributed by major pharmaceutical companies.

Any patient who tells a traditional neurologist that "I'm taking herbs" or "I'm using natural medicines" often gets a stern lecture from the doctor. In keeping with their traditional educations that embrace and advance the objectives of huge pharmaceutical companies— Big Pharma—these physicians usually refer to homeopathy as "quackery."

Such statements often stun, confuse and even mystify patients who often tend to believe what they're told by such professionals. That might seem understandable, since after all, those who lack extensive medical education in our society are expected to follow or believe what they're told by legitimate and certified standard-practice doctors.

These paradoxical situations leave doctors such as me in a quandary. Remember that as an integrative medical oncologist, I practice and embrace both homeopathy and so-called standard-practice medicines.

"Neurologists are flat-out wrong when they tell you that homeopathy is not legitimate," I tell any patient who inquires, particularly those seeking pain relief. "The science and practice of homeopathy serves a vital, urgent and mandatory role in medicine. And any doctor who dares to tell you otherwise is ill-advised and misinformed."

Chapter 35

Homeopathic Pain Therapies Prove Just as Effective

Depending on individual conditions, circumstances and remedies, some natural homeopathic pain remedies are just as effective as expensive pills from Big Pharma.

When I make such irrefutable and well-documented assertions, many physicians and other professionals from standard-practice medicines begin to scoff and whine. Undoubtedly, many standard allopathic doctors fear that natural remedies will endanger their livelihoods. When this happens, are such physicians working in the best interest of patients, or primarily for the doctors' own financial gain?

Some researchers, scientists and standard-medicine doctors might tell you that "homeopathic medicines are only as good as a placebo." These whiners also sometimes proclaim that homeopathic substances lack the "pharmacology" or potency of pharmaceuticals made by the huge drug companies—some costing many dollars per pill.

Yet, I easily could find myself asking such complainers, "Why do you consider the much more costly drug more effective? Could your perception stem from the fact that Big Pharma pills are much more expensive than natural remedies?"

Topping this off, as a highly experienced physician now entering my fifth decade as a practicing physician and now as a registered homeopathic doctor as well, I have witnessed many instances where natural substances worked effectively on pain. This serves as a promising observation, especially because overall the dangerous drugs made by Big Pharma generate far more serious potential side effects.

Some Homeopathic Remedies Do A Good Job Fighting Pain

In some instances the best treatments stem from the remedies embraced or recommended by standard medicines and Big Pharma. Even so, from my perspective common sense dictates that physicians should at least consider the potential remedies proposed by homeopathy, depending on the specific case and the symptoms involved.

Homeopaths choose from a wide range of potential substances for specific ailments, including the alleviation of pain. The many hundreds of options range from various combinations of salts, snake venoms, and thyroid hormone extracts. Some options also include various substances derived from living organisms that are deemed healthy.

Within this branch of medicine, such substances are often referred to as "remedies," although this term should never imply a guaranteed cure or a lessening of symptoms. Meantime, all practicing homeopaths recommend variations of exercise, a healthy diet and good physical hygiene such as cleanliness.

In preparing remedies issued by homeopaths, specific substances often are mixed or diluted with alcohol or distilled water. Some observers or critics point out that the mixing of various substances— sometimes intended for pain—might result in toxic reactions. From my perspective, this is among primary reasons why patients seeking homeopathic treatments should seek the services of only a licensed, highly trained homeopath.

Familiarize Yourself with Top Homeopathic Pain Medicines

While remembering that patients should never attempt to diagnose their own ailments, everyone should feel free to become familiar with some of the top pain-relief remedies used by homeopaths. Among the most common:

- Arnica: Some homeopaths insist this substance often emerges as highly effective in battling the excruciating pains and symptoms of arthritis. Technicians generate "arnica" from an herb, derived from a yellow flower that grows at high elevations in Europe. Patients using arnica usually apply this on the skin in the form of a gel, or orally.

- Curcumin: From the perspective of homeopaths, this helps lessen or prevent painful swelling. The body usually absorbs curcumin better when taken orally as a capsule. Sometimes called "turmeric," curcumin is also used as an anti-inflammatory in battling the potentially crippling symptoms of arthritis. Some patients prefer this to standard medicines for treatments to painful conditions like hemorrhoids.

- Devil's claw: People with pre-existing stomach problems should avoid this often-powerful homeopathic remedy, derived from a fruit that grows in South Africa and often found effective in treatments for everything from backaches to arthritis.

- Feverfew: Homeopaths use this flowering plant prevalent across North America, Europe and the Mediterranean area to generate a medicinal herb—often deemed helpful in generating relief from the pain of headaches and arthritis.

- Frankincense: Perhaps best known worldwide as one of the gifts the three wise kings brought the Infant Jesus along with gold and myrrh, this aromatic resin from the hardy boswellia trees in Armenia is often used in perfumes and even incense. And, besides its use in religious rites, frankincense can be eaten in pure form—a treatment used for hundreds of years for arthritic pain and minor injuries. Some researchers indicate they're studying the possible effects of frankincense on numerous specific painful afflictions, including ulcerative colitis and Crohn's Disease which inflames the intestines.

Varying homeopathic medicines or generalized treatments within this realm have been used for thousands of years, at least according to some published reports. In the late 1700s and early 1800s, the German physician Samuel Hahnemann played an integral role in generating what many people today call "alternative medicine." Even then Hahnemann, the "father of homeopathy," believed that the so-called traditional medicines of his era did "more harm than good."

Chapter 36

Numerous Alternative Medicines Battle Pain

Besides homeopathy, standard or mainstream physicians often frown upon various other alternative medicines. In some instances for thousands of years, many of these diverse and traditional systems have proven effective in eliminating pain or removing the underlying conditions that cause physical discomfort.

From the view of many standard-practice doctors, at least some or perhaps all alternative medicines lack any credible scientific or credible basis. Critics complain that such treatments are not based on credible results from intense, evidence-based research. Nonetheless, countless patients worldwide seem to feel otherwise, seeking treatment and often returning for follow-up checkups, treatments, herbs or therapy sessions. Among just some of the many widely recognized alternative medical practices:

- Naturopathy: Sometimes called naturopathic medicine, these treatments appreciate and recognize that the body possesses an innate ability for self-healing. Practitioners of naturopathy strive to minimize surgeries, while concentrating on a whole-body or "holistic" approach dealing with everything from the patient's mental, physical, bodily and mental conditions, perspectives or environments. Patients often are instructed to undergo a wide range of medicines and lifestyle choices, which can include a variety of exercises, herbs, nutritional objectives, stress reduction methods and acupuncture. Some professional practitioners of naturopathy employ a degree of traditional medicine in their overall approach to fighting pain, while others prefer to employ more alternative strategies such as those often used by homeopaths.

• Herbalism: This specialty concentrates on a vast array of natural-grown plants and herbs that are extracts from plants. Also, some products or substances prescribed by herbalists include substances derived from animals or insects, such as bee venom or specific types of fungus. The many herbs and plant derivatives for fighting pain include meadowsweet, a perennial herb found naturally in Asia and Europe; this has salicylic acid—heralded for its ability to fight pain, reduce fever and relieve inflammation. Other natural pain relievers include plants found on Caribbean and Pacific islands, and a perennial flowering plant found in North America, Asia and Europe, "stinging nettle." More than 120 plants or herbs used in herbalism also are used in making drugs produced by Big Pharma, including some pain killers, according to a 2001 article, "The Value of Plants Used in Traditional Medicine for Drug Discovery."

• Meditation: Embracing traditions and methods used for thousands of years, people who meditate in many cultures strive to put their minds into a specific mode of consciousness—all in efforts to achieve certain benefits, such as the elimination of their own pain. Practitioners of meditation view the mind as a powerful force capable of focusing upon or ignoring physical or mental sensations.

Those who meditate use a variety of methods to achieve the mental state they seek, such as the concentration on compassionate thoughts or the noticing of a specific "focal point." Many branches of meditation stem from ancient Eastern religions or traditions such as Buddhism or Hinduism. According to the "Clinical guide to the treatment of human stress response" published in 2002, in some clinical settings people have used meditation to relieve pain and stress.

- Chiropractic Medicine: Although labeled as "quackery" by some standard-practice doctors, this longtime and widely accepted branch of medicine has been hailed by many patients as effective in fighting severe pain such as backaches or joint aches. Following extensive education in their crafts, doctors of chiropractic excel in diagnosing and treating problems with the body's musculoskeletal system, particularly the spine. Such professionals realize that the spine plays an integral role in the body's nervous system, particularly the integral and highly complex natural system of experiencing pain. Some scientists label chiropractic as an alternative or "complimentary" branch of medicine, separate but potentially related to so-called primary care physicians. When viewed in this regard, chiropractors practice falls within a medical specialty like dentists or podiatrists. Some chiropractors specialize primarily in adjustments of the spine, while others concentrate on that as well while also seeking to mix a variety of other treatments such as herbal supplements or homeopathy.

- Acupuncture: Often in an effort to relieve pain, these highly trained professionals follow the ancient Chinese-based tradition and method of inserting and manipulating needles into specific regions of a patient's body. It is often effectively used in anesthesia. Besides pain relief, acupuncture strives to treat or prevent disease, in addition to the use as a therapy or to strive for good overall health. The methods and concepts embraced by acupuncturists often differ from the scientific-based strategies and diagnosis methods accepted by traditional doctors. Acupuncture emerged in prehistoric times, thousands of years before the advent of cellular theory, complex discoveries in biology and integral research into the human anatomy. Even after such scientific medical advances, many patients worldwide have sworn to what they call the great and reliable effectiveness of acupuncture. Also, acupuncture points are directly related to internal organ systems.

- Biofeedback: Modern-day science-based devices are attached to patients, who can then continuously monitor their own vital signs—everything from the heart rate and breathing rates to muscle tension, brainwaves and skin temperature. According to some published reports, biofeedback has proven effective in treating headaches and migraines as patients use the monitors while teaching themselves to relax, breathe slowly and to control their own sensations of pain.

- Lamaze: This is among numerous natural childbirth techniques that teach women various methods of coping with extreme pain during labor—without resorting to traditional standard-medicine drugs to relieve pain. Lamaze is among natural birthing systems that some critics claim lacks any evidence-based proof that it works as an effective medical therapy. Nonetheless, many Lamaze proponents embrace and encourage this method, which entails everything from learning to breathe through the pain to massage and spontaneous pushing. Proponents of natural childbirth methods such as Lamaze proclaim this process hails as the healthy and much-preferred alternative to mainstream medical techniques. Many women who chose to give birth naturally fear that local anesthetics sometimes used by traditional mainstream physicians might pose potential harm to themselves or to their babies. Proponents of natural childbirth argue that women are biologically capable of giving birth without medical assistance.

- Hypnosis: Just about anyone who has seen a hypnotist perform live on stage, on TV or in the movies realizes that this system strives to control the brain's reactions, thoughts or perceptions. While many people and especially mainstream physicians consider hypnosis as "pure quackery," a hypnotist strives to control the mind of a person. And, sometimes an individual tries to control his or her own brain process through "self-hypnosis." Practitioners of hypnosis claim that for the most part people who willingly get hypnotized often respond readily to suggestions—either physically or psychologically. While the process is actually quite complex, hypnotists strive verbally and non-verbally to focus the person's conscious mind on a single predominant objective or idea in order to make the individual more susceptible to suggestions. Basically, the underlying core of hypnosis is "mind control," a highly controversial topic for a variety of obvious reasons. Meantime, battling pain remains among this system's potential objectives.

Besides these systems along with homeopathy and ancient Chinese medicine, people worldwide seek help from pain from a vast range of other alternative medicines. These include traditional therapies, plus medical disciplines from specific cultures or nations such as Tibet and Mongolia.

In fact, literally hundreds of alternative medicine structures or philosophies still exist, such as intentional fasting, faith healing, the intentional drinking of urine, using magnets for therapy, and countless others that I would rarely recommend—if ever. Nonetheless, an age-old American proverb proclaims that "variety is the spice of life." Such zest and vibrancy within our mainstream medical culture is needed to give everyone a pathway to getting much-needed relief from pain. For those seeking any potential alternative medicine to relieve pain, I recommend that the person conduct extensive research before seeking such options.

Chapter 37

Physical Therapy Also Plays a Vital Role in Fighting Pain

Besides good nutrition, exercise and the administering of specific drugs or remedies, the process of physical therapy plays a vital and essential role in the fight against pain. Those who undergo physical therapies range from people injured in accidents to those who suffered strokes, severe illness or chronic ailments.

Conducted by certified physical therapists, this primary health care process strives to enable people to regain or retain their abilities to move their bodies in a natural, functional way. Physical therapy can help improve posture and also boost overall health, thereby potentially lessening or eliminating pain.

Patients who undergo physical therapy often are encouraged to make such efforts a lifelong process. This stems largely from a continual need to remain vigilant at striving to move, walk or pick up objects in natural ways, even amid persistent and chronic ailments, advanced age, or certain irreversible after-effects from injuries.

The process of re-learning to move certain ways or improving muscular functions via physical therapy can help improve bodily functions and the psyche as well. Such improvements sometimes generate more positive attitudes in patients, sparking or re-energizing motivations that enable them to battle their own physical discomforts.

Many certified and much-respected specialties of physical therapy target everything from neurology and pediatrics to centers for cardiopulmonary patients and facilities focusing on the unique needs of senior citizens.

Starting with hydrotherapy, message and manual therapy nearly 500 years before Christ, the earliest physicians of the Greek culture including Hippocrates reportedly began to recognize the value of continually attempting to resume body movements. Physical therapies blossomed in the late 1800s in Britain. The process soon spread to America, where remedial exercise increased as an important aspect of such treatments.

This field of medicine surged amid the polio outbreak of 1916, followed soon afterward by World War I when physicians began recruiting nurses to assist wounded soldiers in active efforts to regain their abilities to move in natural ways.

Today, the many neurological disorders or functions targeted by specific physical therapies include such painful or debilitating conditions as stroke, Parkinson's Disease, brain injuries, cerebral palsy, and joint replacements such as the hip.

Anyone now fighting painful conditions while suffering from physical disabilities should ask a certified medical professional whether physical therapy might help eliminate pain. Some medical insurance plans cover most costs for such treatments.

"Depending on your individual circumstance, physical therapy might go a long way in enabling you to battle pain," I tell some patients, especially those who inquire. "The best way to determine that possibility is to first conduct a complete diagnosis, and then we'll take it from there."

Exercise or Physical Therapy Go A Long Way in Battling Pain

Needless to say, physical exercise boosts the immune system while improving bodily functions such as muscular tone and bone strength. These functions can go a long way toward preventing or lessening the probability of painful conditions. Meantime, these overall improvements in the patient's ability to move or lift objects can enable the individual to recover more rapidly from illness or injury, particularly if extensive and regular exercise begins well beforehand.

Athletic coaches and military generals have known for many generations that their athletes or soldiers who have well-conditioned bodies have decreased chances of injuries and an improved likelihood of quick recoveries if physical problems should occur.

Besides honing their mental skills and fine-tuning the abilities to conform to rules or necessary skill-sets, well-conditioned soldiers and athletes reportedly have faster and better mental reactions in challenging and potentially dangerous situations. Such high-level mental functioning can increase the person's ability to escape painful results.

In both military and sports settings, well conditioned bodies also can increase the likelihood of victory for the entire team. While going a long way to battle or prevent potentially painful outcomes, this philosophy of excellent physical conditioning often spills over into the important professions of firefighters, police officers and prison personnel.

Chapter 38

Discover the Rapidly Expanding Pain Management Industry

Boosted by rapid advances in medical technology and improved therapies, physicians, hospitals and related professionals are banding together to develop collective systems—working en masse to fight the pain of individual patients. In recent years, this steadily evolving process has been coined as "pain management."

Certainly, from my view this collective process in joining forces for the betterment of patients makes good sense. Interdisciplinary medical professionals work together or communicate en tandem to generate a prognosis and to develop treatments for each patient's pain.

With a collective goal of improving each patient's quality of life, professionals who join pain management teams sometimes include everyone from standard-practice physicians, clinical psychologists and nurse practitioners to occupational therapists.

In some patients, pain disappears or at least subsides after physical therapy or medicines helps eliminate or lessen the medical problem that causes their discomfort. When a patient's pain persists due to trauma, illness or any pathological condition such as arthritis, the person sometimes gets targeted for help from a pain management team.

Depending on specific circumstances, some treatments delve into the psychological realm of what physicians call "cognitive behavioral therapy." This specific branch usually entails working to resolve apparent or possible problems with the person's emotions and behaviors.

Besides the possibility of using anesthesiologists and neurologists, the many other professionals on pain management teams might also include psychiatrists. Working collectively and individually in recommending or prescribing treatments, such experts can employ a vast array of therapies or drugs. These range from inserting drugs directly into the spinal cord or brain in an "intrathecal" process, using spinal cord stimulators to send electrical pulses into that organ, epidural steroid injections, and many other options.

Physicians Disable the Spinal Cord in Extreme Cases of Pain

Certain severe, excruciatingly painful medical instances motivate physicians to undertake the extraordinary procedure of disabling sections of the spinal cord. Specifically, this process called a "cordotomy" involves a surgical procedure where specific pain-conducting tracts within the spinal cord are disabled.

In layman's terms, the cordotomy procedures are usually done as a last resort in cases where a patient is terminally ill with inoperable afflictions such as highly advanced prostate cancer, or for a variety of incurable diseases.

Such specific and complex surgeries, often performed as a humanitarian measure to relieve a patient of extreme pain during life's final stage, usually are performed with a needle rather than by opening the body with a scalpel. During a cordotomy, the patient usually does not feel pain in the area of the operation thanks to a local anesthetic.

Amid the procedure, the surgeon often uses a fluoroscopy device that enables the viewing of the body's internal structures. However, the procedure poses potential risks, primarily because in certain instances the patient gets exposed to consistent but low doses of radiation—a known carcinogen.

Before undergoing a cordotomy the physician strives to consider the risks to the patient when matched to the urgent need to eliminate pain—plus the person's overall current condition. Also, for the most part, physicians usually recommend a cordotomy to a patient only after treatments in the highest level of the ladder of pain, primarily opium-derived drugs, have failed to get adequate results.

Some Procedures Even Involve the Removal of Nerves

Other high-level, final-resort procedures to eliminate excruciating and chronic pain sometimes involve what doctor's call "nerve ablation"—literally the removal of that organ from the body. Most ablations involve procedures that do not attempt to relieve pain, such as facelifts or the removal of wrinkled skin, or even deadening certain areas of the atria via electrical frequencies in attempts to abolish abnormal heartbeats.

When targeting pain, the nerve ablation process can entail removing a specific wounded or damaged area of the body, or taking out a section of the brain that senses the discomfort. Some neurological disorders such as Parkinson's disease sometimes result in doctors recommending the removal of certain areas of the brain.

Much of the time the ablation of nerves or tumors is done via lasers with varying degrees of intensity. While minimally invasive to the body, such procedures are sometimes called "radio frequency ablation."

In addition to the removal of small-sized body parts or nerves in efforts to eliminate pain, doctors also sometimes must resort to the amputation of entire limbs. Amputations are usually done only in extreme cases, not usually for the specific purpose of relieving pain, but primarily due to the deadening, or to an extreme and irreversible disfiguring of the limb.

Eager to add much-needed humor to the process, some patients might refer to their "previous amputations," such as the necessary removal of an entire pain-causing body through the process of divorce. Certainly, the removal of any part of the human body is no cause for open humor among medical professionals. But since the very thought and notion of such procedures can generate a depressing mood, a little levity can go a long way in helping the patient pick up his or her spirits.

Major Strides Against Pain Developed in the Wars in Iraq and Afghanistan

The concept and process of pain management has jumped into full-speed, thanks to major advances developed by U.S. military medical personnel amid the wars in Iraq and Afghanistan. Doctors, scientists and medical-based corporations have worked together to develop quick therapeutic and pain-relieving processes for our wounded troops.

Caught in the line of fire, these tried-and-true battlefield techniques have enabled military commanders to develop a system where severely wounded troops are extracted from battlefields as soon as possible. From there, our soldiers often are in operating rooms within a half hour after suffering horrendous injuries, many of their wounds life-threatening.

Working together, expert medical crews strive as soon as possible to restore each wounded soldier's vital signs as soon as possible to optimal levels. Meantime, the soldiers in the battle zones and medical crews make the elimination of pain a top priority.

Streams of news reports in recent years have chronicled how these loyal and dedicated professionals have strived to bring relief to their comrades, who often suffer from extreme physical and emotional pain during recuperation. One of the most publicized cases involved Bob Woodruff, former anchor of the ABC-TV's "World News Tonight."

Doctors quickly performed an emergency surgery on Woodruff's skull and brain shortly after a roadside bomb in Iraq exploded in January 2006. A Canadian cameraman also was wounded in the same attack. The story of Woodruff's recovery is just one of many hundreds of instances where today's military has used the lessons learned in previous wars as a basis for assisting our soldiers wounded in these political hotspots.

According to some news reports, at least 35,000 of the 1.65 million U.S. military service personnel deployed to Iraq and Afghanistan have been physically wounded. The advent and continued development of pain management teams should go a long way in addressing their physical and emotional pains. Meantime, extraordinary advancements have been made in the development of prosthetics.

The Wars Expanded Addictions to Pain Killing Drugs

Despite the admirable advancements our military has made in the fight against physical pain, many of our soldiers, sailors and Air Force personnel have developed extreme addictions to the medications designed to fight such discomfort.

In January 2011, "USA Today" reported that one of our nations's most respected and highest-decorated three-star generals, Lt. Gen. David Fridovich, publicly admitted to his troops of his own extreme addiction to pain killers. Standing before more than 700 of his personnel, Fridovich courageously admitted to his personal mistakes in this regard; he urged the troops to use caution when administering pain killers to our military personnel.

In a front-page article, the newspaper described how the general had been quietly hooked on pain killers during the previous five years. And, the story said, hospitalizations and diagnosis for substance abuse has doubled among members of the armed forces during the past decade. In fact, according to another "USA Today" article published the same day, from 25 percent to 35 percent of the 10,000 military personnel assigned to "wounded care companies or battalions are addicted to or dependant on drugs."

Such news comes as a sad, tragic development, especially to the many medical professionals—inside and outside of our military—who strive daily to legitimately and effectively eliminate the physical pains of others.

As a Vietnam Veteran and a retired U.S. Army National Guard Colonel, I applaud, admire and appreciate the courageous and admirable service of our troops in the Middle East and South Asia. Yet, just like Gen. Fridovich had, I believe that our military can and should do more to confront and address the nagging problems of pain killer addictions among our troops.

First, the military should implement a better "command and control system" that involves the distribution and prescribing of pain killers. And second, the military also should implement the use of well-controlled and carefully monitored natural human growth hormones, in order to speed up the natural healing process and thereby eliminate pain.

Chapter 39

Stop Ignoring and Start Using Human Growth Hormones

As described in my hot-selling book "Anti-Aging Cures," with superstar media personality Suzanne Somers writing the foreword, natural human growth hormones are an effective way to slow down the signs of aging—and for speeding up the natural healing process as well.

For those who have not yet read that publication, in summary, human growth hormone—sometimes called HGH—is produced within the brain. This sparks the continual growth process in children, progressing until their early adult years in their mid-20s. After that age, the body's natural production of HGH steadily slows and people begin to show the signs of aging, such as wrinkles, weight gain and the weakening of bones.

When we're young, though, high levels of HGH that are bodies naturally generate, most often while we sleep, enable us to recover and heal rapidly from wounds and broken bones. Yet older people generally do not recover from such maladies as quickly as the very young, primarily due to the body's steady decrease in production of the hormone after age 25.

This is where the controversy erupts. You see, much of the general public wrongly believes that HGH is illegal. To the contrary, within the United States, the substance is legal when prescribed by a certified medical professional after first conducting a physical examination, and ordering the appropriate tests.

When used properly, HGH can go a long way toward rapidly speeding up the healing process and thereby removing pain—even among our younger wounded soldiers who already naturally produce the hormone at a fairly strong pace. The misconception about HGH stems largely from its abuse in professional sports. Journalists often give HGH an unnecessary and unwarranted bad rap.

Make HGH More Widely Accessible

To heal wounds faster and thereby accelerate the natural decrease in pain, hospital emergency rooms nationwide and around the world need to make HGH more readily available to victims of accidents and extreme trauma such as gunshot wounds.

Since HGH reigns as a naturally occurring and vital biological substance, administering this hormone under proper conditions at recommended doses—but not in excessive amounts—should evolve into a preferred and logical alternative. This should become an accepted, logical potential alternative to some unnatural, highly dangerous and expensive medications that generate giant profits for "Big Pharma," the large pharmaceutical companies.

As a licensed homeopath and a seasoned oncologist and physician, I have witnessed many instances where standard, mainstream doctors ignore the natural substances such as HGH—even though this hormone can go a long way in the battle of fighting pain.

Sadly, however, many standard allopathic doctors are trained to do

302

only what they're taught, which often means avoiding any natural treatments that would enable patients to heal the way that nature intended.

As a society, our entire culture needs to do more to accept and generate natural substances such as HGH, largely because they're far less expensive than many high-end pharmaceuticals while often proving more effective than potentially dangerous drugs issued and promoted by Big Pharma.

Chapter 40

Corruption in Third World Countries and Other Nations Compounds the Problem

Greedy medical professionals in countries outside North America are compounding the problem, in conjunction with money-hungry U.S.-based drug companies.

An increasingly steady number of news reports in recent years have described how low-paid doctors in countries such as China over-prescribe pain drugs and antibiotic medications. According to a February 2011 article in "USA Today," this problem occurs because the compensation for usually low-paid doctors in China is based on how much revenue they generate.

As a result, in an effort to increase their own pay, many of these physicians sometimes issue pain medications or other drugs delivered via IV drips, although in many cases these treatments are unnecessary. Compounding the problems, according the article, pharmaceutical companies sometimes issue kickbacks to low-paid Chinese doctors who are willing to issue prescriptions for the corporation's drugs.

Adding more heartache to this corrupt system, some unsuspecting patients who receive pain killers and other drugs experience severe overdoses and critical medical complications. Across China and numerous other nations where entire societies are just beginning to benefit from advancements in medical technology, the responsibility goes to "barefoot doctors"—such as farmers who once learned the rudimentary basics of medicine.

On an international scale, the overall ongoing battle by the entire human population in fighting physical pain is complex, corrupt and failing patients in many societies.

As a result, I strongly urge physicians everywhere and especially the large drug companies to work primarily in the best interest of each patient. Doctors everywhere need to remind themselves to adhere to the Hippocratic Oath, which all physicians take when entering the profession, promising to practice medicine in an ethical manner.

Far from being a holier-than-thou statement on my part, such mindful and clear-cut objectives should remain at the forefront of physicians everywhere. This adherence to a supreme ethical standard also should hold fast throughout the upcoming advancements in pain-fighting technology.

People Everywhere Demand Improved Health Care

In recent years people from many nations worldwide have been rioting in the streets of their countries, demanding the formation and implementation of democratic governments. Many of these complaints stem from a basic desire for more personal freedom and better services, particularly in the arena of better health care in the fight against pain and the various ailments that cause such discomfort.

As democracy evolves and spreads in these numerous nations, let us hope that any new or emerging governments clear the way for more advanced and competitive medical systems. Hopefully, such improvements in infrastructure will start benefiting more people, rather than just those lucky enough to live in the world's wealthiest countries.

Meantime, here in the United States, individual consumers need to demand that their hospitals and doctors adhere to the highest possible ethical standards in developing and implementing superior pain medications and physical therapies.

Thanks largely to the Human Genome Project, let us all hope for amazing technological advancements in fighting pain in the near future. Until such developments click into gear, we all need to remain vigilant in monitoring and reporting the progress of these vital and urgent advancements.

To help put this overall situation into basic, easy-to-understand "human terms" that almost anyone can comprehend, I like to point out that the 1990s and the first decade of this century became the catalyst era for vital digital technologies such as the Internet and cell phones. I predict that in much the same way the medical field will develop significant, life-changing advancements during the 2010s and 2020s.

As the living world population tips the 7 billion mark, we all need to keep in mind that a vast majority of these individuals will eventually suffer severe pains—particularly as they mature, long past the age of 25 when the human body peaks in its natural production of HGH.

In much the way that Viagra® and similar drugs turned the world upside down so to speak with the advent of medication to correct the adverse symptoms of male erectile dysfunction, the international community is likely to find itself startled and amazed when scientists create an all-new, non-addictive and highly potent pain medication.

The pharmaceutical company or clinic that develops this "miracle drug" is likely to emerge as a big winner—deserving the thanks of all humanity. Until that occurs, however, we should all collectively seek the least addictive, most powerful treatments possible while progressing to more potent and addictive drugs only when necessary.

Unethical Sales of Pain Pills Erupted in Controversy

The controversy of painkillers skyrocketed into a fever pitch in February 2011, when police and federal agents barged into the South Florida offices of doctors suspected of over-prescribing highly addictive pain killers like Oxycodone.

Authorities seized literally dozens of exotic cars in the raids, which resulted in the arrests of at least 22 people including physicians. The U.S. Drug Enforcement Agency, commonly called the "DEA," joined police in calling the operations "pill mills."

Any suspects, of course, were presumed innocent until such time as they might be proven guilty. Meantime, I became among many physicians numbed by the thought that other licensed doctors would intentionally over-prescribe such highly addictive drugs.

While authorities allege such illegal operations thrive nationwide, these enterprises have excelled at an astounding rate across Florida far more than any other state. Various news media reports said that purchases of oxycodone in Florida surpassed the purchases of the same drug in all states combined during the first half of 2010. Amazingly, however, Florida was among states that lack programs to monitor these pervasive drug pipelines; the Sunshine State's Republican governor at the time, Rick Scott, had been quoted as saying that such an effort would be too expensive and an invasion of privacy.

Investigators claim that operators of these cash-only clinics conducted only cursory medical examinations, before the facilities' physicians issued prescriptions for narcotic pain killers. A DEA spokesman, Rusty Payne, told "USA Today" in a front-page article that some clinics had in-house pharmacies to fill the prescriptions, which included such highly addictive substances as oxycodone and hydrocodone.

Boosted in part by strong new state laws forbidding such drug distribution systems, authorities have done a commendable job in launching the nationwide crackdown on pill mills and the doctors who profit from them. Even so, far more needs to be done in order to clamp down on this increasingly complex and pervasive problem. Among my primary suggestions, which mirror those of many top officials including the nation's drug czar, Gil Kerlikowske:

- Databases: The various states need to jointly start and operate a database, in order to pinpoint and target any doctor who over-prescribes pain killers, and also to identify and target patients who seek excessive amounts of such prescriptions.

- New Legislation: The legislatures of some states including Florida should go ahead with plans already submitted by some lawmakers, requiring that any patient who receives such drugs first undergo examinations by doctors at pain clinics.

- Increase Penalties: Intensify and tighten the proverbial noose, making $10,000 fines and six-month suspensions mandatory for physicians found guilty of over-prescribing such medications.

- Doctor Shopping: Use the information from the database to prevent attempts by patients to obtain multiple prescriptions for pain medications in numerous states. Meantime, a handful of states already have programs to monitor such prescriptions, including Kentucky and Tennessee.

Despite these primary regulations already either proposed or suggested by various officials, our leaders need to do much more to slam down on Big Pharma, which makes no significant effort whatsoever to limit these over-prescriptions. Instead of just blaming doctors and patients, authorities need to tighten their grips on the free-flowing and unchecked distribution of harmful pain killers to the pill mills.

Why Do Efforts Fail to Regulate the Flow of Pain Killers?

News reports indicate many doctors are willing to issue unnecessary pain killer prescriptions due to plain old fashioned greed. This situation worsens when factoring in extreme problems for society and to the individuals involved.

Various journalists and publications claim that the abuse of prescription drugs—primarily pain killers—afflict at least 7 million people nationwide of age 12 and older. If true, this would make such addictions the third most widely abused drugs in the United States, behind alcohol and marijuana.

Greedy drug pushers and money-hungry doctors who issue too many pain killer prescriptions know that for just more than a few hundred bucks, patients at pill mills or who receive unnecessary prescriptions from standard physicians can get about 100 pills. Those same drugs obtained on the legitimate market are sometimes then sold by the gram, with a street value of about $5,400, experts say.

Ultimately, the very essence of Mother Nature requires that human beings suffer physical pain. And, thankfully, our creator generated the ideal plants and substances such as willow tree bark and even opium to fight or remove such sensations. Yet herein rests a "rub," a horrible paradox because those very drugs intended to help people often end up destroying many lives.

Besides ravaging the finances of entire families, prescription-level pain killer narcotics damage and permanently wreck the minds and bodies of those suffering the highest levels of abuse. Many of the most frequently abused drugs fall within the realm of high-level analgesics at least to some degree, ranging from psychoactive drugs to performance enhancing narcotics.

Once again, keep in mind that substances in the psychoactive class alter everything from mood and levels of consciousness to behavior

311

and even the ability to assimilate information. And, as you've already learned, drugs within the performance-enhancing class include highly dangerous anabolic steroids.

Taken individually or in mixtures of various substances, these many drugs slam deep into the lives and families of those who get hooked. Spouses and children of the primary drug abuser often suffer, especially when finances get depleted, the addict suffers physical and mental deterioration, and relatives feel hopeless in efforts to save their loved ones from permanent physical and mental degradation.

Besides long-term heartlessness toward their relatives, many drug abusers commit robberies, burglaries and assaults in efforts to get money necessary to feed their habits.

Primarily for these reasons, we all need to remain cognizant of the potential extreme dangers of such drugs. When and if you legally take such substances under a physician's care, follow instructions carefully and strive from the start to avoid becoming addicted. And, if you, a loved one, friend or acquaintance shows early signs of such behavior, strive to seek professional help as soon as possible.

Al Capone, a notorious Chicago mobster and bootlegger during the Roaring '20s prohibition era when alcohol was legally banned, once said that "When I sell liquor, it's called bootlegging. When my patrons serve it on Lake Short Drive, it's called hospitality."

Sure enough, when personal matters involve alcohol and particular pain killers, many of us tend to rationalize the situation. Such individuals think: "Serious pain-killer addiction cannot happen to me. I can never become addicted, and in fact, I'm not addicted at this time. I just take these drugs like I'm doing now for an important personal medical condition."

James W. Forsythe, M.D., H.M.D.

Never Legalize Highly Powerful Pain Killers

Using arguments that I personally find bizarre and convoluted, some people proclaim that narcotics and especially pain killers should be legalized. These individuals insist that our prisons are clogged with drug abusers and distributors, but that public resources would be better used in the rehabilitation process outside of penitentiaries.

Proponents of legalized substance abuse, such as the late "tune-in, turn-on, and drop-out" advocate Timothy Leary, have insisted that drugs of many kinds have proven relatively harmless when legally administered to entire societies. From this way of thinking, at least to a degree, the abuse of illegal substances has been equated to the prohibition era when the U.S. government outlawed the production, distribution and sale of alcohol.

Herein rests and extraordinary and pivotal question: Would legalizing narcotics cut down on crime, abuse, excessive and extraordinarily high "street prices" for narcotics—while also alleviating prison overcrowding? Would legalizing the distribution and sale of extremely strong painkillers such as morphine, opium and heroin lessen the great potential harm posed by such substances on all of society?

Without question, these are pivotal and integral dilemmas that face almost the entire world, especially as national, state, provincial and local governments struggle with increasingly problematic budget crises.

With luck, researchers will develop a reliable, indisputable and 100-percent effective non-addictive pain killer—perhaps thanks largely to the Human Genome Project. For the time being, however, the probability of whether scientists can develop such a medication remains only a mere possibility.

When and if such advancement finally occurs, with luck authorities worldwide could then destroy all opium plants and other substances. This could potentially eliminate at least a great number of the many specific types of addictions to pain killers.

Yet, in the big scope of things, I find this situation almost impossible. After all, why would greedy pharmaceutical companies ever entertain the very notion of cutting off a huge hunk of their own stranglehold on the pernicious multi-billion-dollar mainstream drug industry?

While society remains saddled with all these many dilemmas, at least one thing remains certain. In all likelihood human beings will continue to experience physical pains through the end of this century and perhaps even for hundreds or thousands of years. For as long as mankind continues to thrive and prosper, people will continue to suffer from these physical sensations. Otherwise, people of both genders and of all races and cultures would fail to notice and eventually treat their own illnesses and injuries.

To be sure, the evolution of pain management is likely to continue evolving as a unique and integral aspect of what some sociologists call the "human experiment." As the many advancement and positive developments in the ongoing battle against pain continues in the coming decades, scientists and doctors should have plenty of good news to announce.

Take Decisive Action When Battling Your Pain

Like I've said, every week patients from around the world visit my West Coast clinic in the United States to continue their battles against cancer and other physically painful conditions.

I encourage them to ask me as many questions as possible about the many potential ways to eliminate or lessen their bodily discomforts. Many want to know more about the natural alternatives, while others prefer to focus on so-called mainstream options. For each patient, of course, I only make recommendations or issue prescriptions and treatments after conducting a thorough medical examination and reaching a prognosis.

Perhaps my popularity among patients stems largely from word-of-mouth, such as those video proclamations many of them have made for my Website—DrForsythe.com. And, of course, I'm told that the increasing popularity of my books and those written about me play a huge role in attracting patients.

Many of my patients and work associates tell me they're amazed at my continued stamina although I'm now edging into my mid-70s. Unlike many successful doctors who only work three or four days weekly during the final stage of their careers, I work a minimum of five days weekly and sometimes much more. The stream of new patients at my clinic has intensified and increased markedly in recent years. All along, my drive and passion for the medical profession continues to blossom and increase more than ever before.

Maybe this stems in part from the fact that I practice what I preach, so to speak. And I exercise and eat healthy foods for the most part, a process that I recommend for all my patients in order to achieve or maintain good health—the desired physical condition that goes a long way in preventing painful diseases or injuries. In addition, I take daily supplements for my heart, prostate, cholesterol and immune system to fortify myself.

Ask Lots of Questions and Find the Right Doctors

Anyone suffering from extreme pain, or their conscious and caring relatives, should ask as many questions as possible when interacting with their doctors or medical professionals. You should always ask why specific procedures or medications are recommended, and for details on potential adverse side effects.

Just as important, remember to inquire about any viable natural alternatives, and even if such substances are possible to deaden severe pain without your having to resort to powerful, highly addictive opium-based pharmaceuticals.

Also, remember that when dealing solely with mainstream physicians, you're likely to hear that natural healing methods or alternative medicines are nothing but "quackery." All along, even if given such negative statements, you should remain inquisitive and keep an open mind about your options.

From my way of thinking, if any mainstream doctor ever tells you that there is no hope for eliminating your physical pain other than via extremely dangerous drugs, you should actively seek or consider a variety of other options as well.

Certainly, no person should have to endure chronic physical pain, especially if such a condition might prevent the person from enjoying at least a basic, sensible and fairly good quality of life. Ultimately, there are numerous highly effective options that you can always seek, but such remedies should be sought only under the continual monitoring and guidance of a licensed medical professional.

As Johann Wolfgang von Goethe, the German novelist once proclaimed: "We are forced to participate in the games of life before we can possibly learn how to use the options in the rules governing them." Indeed you should let your body's physical reactions to the various therapies, medications and treatments serve as your guide— potentially inspiring you to seek other options or treatments when current attempts to relieve your pain seem fruitless.

About the Author

James W. Forsythe, M.D., H.M.D., is an author, anti-aging physician, and integrative medical oncologist specializing in the use of human growth hormone to combat the symptoms of aging. A native of Detroit, Michigan, Forsythe has won widespread acclaim for his many medical achievements in the battles against cancer. Details on Doctor Forsythe's medical practice and on his numerous books can be found at his Website, DrForsythe.com

Other Books by the Author

"Anti-Aging Cures"
Discover risks and rewards,
of everything from diets to toxins

For complete and in-depth details on following these good lifestyle paths, get Dr. Forsythe's book,

"Anti-Aging Cures"
The book describes in detail why we age, plus a variety of methods to safely delay or stall signs of the body's maturing process—everything from wrinkles to excess body fat. To maintain good health or to put yourself on track for recovery, Dr. Forsythe's book teaches the intricacies of everything from vitamins and diet, to appropriate exercise habits and even toxins that you should avoid. Suzanne Somers wrote the foreward for **"Anti-Aging Cures, Discover risks and rewards, of everythng from diets to toxins"** book and is being promoted by her.

Books written or co-written by Dr. Forsythe

Suzanne Somers' number one best sellers:

"KNOCKOUT, Interviews with Doctors Who Are Curing Cancer"
and "BREAKTHROUGH, Eight Steps To Wellness "

"An Alternative Medicine Definitive Guide to Cancer"

continued on next page

"The Ultimate Guide To Natural Health, Quick Reference A-Z Directory
of Natural Remedies for Diseases and Ailments"

"The Healing Power of Sleep"

"Sleep and Grow Young... With the Magic of REM"

and

"Emergency Radiation Medical Handbook
The Essential, Mandatory Guide for Citizens and Responders
to Nuclear Events"

James W. Forsythe, M.D., H.M.D

Diplomate of the Specialty Board of Medical Oncology
American Board of Internal Medicine
Certified in Homeopathy

Office: 775-827-0707
1-877-789-0707
Fax: 775-827-1006

521 Hammill Lane
Reno, NV 89511

www.centurywellness.com

www.DrForsythe.com